Building Communication and Independence
for Children Across the Autism Spectrum

Building Communication and Independence for Children Across the Autism Spectrum

Strategies to Address Minimal Language, Echolalia and Behavior

Elizabeth Ives Field

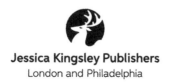

Jessica Kingsley Publishers
London and Philadelphia

First published in Great Britain in 2021 by Jessica Kingsley Publishers
An Hachette Company

2

Copyright © Elizabeth Ives Field 2021

A CIP catalogue record for this title is available from the British Library and the Library of Congress

ISBN 978 1 78775 546 8
eISBN 978 1 78775 547 5

Printed and bound in Great Britain by Clays Ltd, Elcograf S.p.A.

Jessica Kingsley Publishers' policy is to use papers that are natural, renewable and recyclable
products and made from wood grown in sustainable forests. The logging and manufacturing
processes are expected to conform to the environmental regulations of the country of origin.

Jessica Kingsley Publishers
73 Collier Street
London N1 9BE, UK

www.jkp.com

With gratitude for the many children, teens and families who have shared their autism journeys with me. Without them, my life would be less rich and there would be no book.

Acknowledgements

My first and biggest thank you goes to my dear friend and colleague, Gail Tudor. She read the whole manuscript multiple times as it developed and provided much guidance and support. Two recurring themes were, "That's an awfully long sentence with too much jammed into it" and "Well, I know what you mean here, but your reader might not." Because of Gail's involvement, the writing process was a lot more fun and the product is undoubtedly better.

I am also grateful to these other friends, family and colleagues who have read parts of the book and offered encouragement and suggestions along the way: Kelly Field Green, Gayle Flegel, Shawn Gillespie, Jane Ives, Lori Spencer, Beverly Stessel, Samuel Stessel and Ann Weston.

And I appreciate the support, camaraderie and suggestions from my friends in the writers' groups at the public libraries of Hudson and Sudbury, Massachusetts.

Thank you to the team at Jessica Kingsley Publishers who have nurtured my book and cheerfully guided me into the fascinating world of publishing. Special thanks to my editor, Sarah Hamlin, for her advocacy, advice and answers.

Contents

Part III   Advanced Language with Gaps

Some Notes

Person-first or identity-first?

There is some controversy in the international autism community over the use of person-first or identity-first language. Should we refer to a "child with autism" (person-first) or an "autistic child" (identity-first)?

Some parents have a strong preference for person-first language and many professionals have been instructed to use it always.

Some adults with autism spectrum diagnoses strongly prefer to be known as autistic adults while others, like my friend Samuel, consider the controversy to be a distraction from more important issues.

Either way, we are discussing unique individuals with some shared challenges. I am comfortable with either terminology and you will find both person-first and identity-first language in this book. I hope this compromise will be acceptable to my readers.

Pseudonyms

The children and teens described in this book all have invented names and their characteristics are based on several people who have had similar needs and abilities.

Pronouns

I do not like to keep repeating "he or she" and I will bet that you don't like reading it either. Because four times as many boys as girls are diagnosed with autism (American Psychiatric Association 2013, p.57), I default to the male pronouns most often when describing characteristics of groups. However, there certainly are girls on the autism spectrum. They are important, and whole books have been written about them. Here, they and their female pronouns will be represented in two of the nine case descriptions.

References

References used or mentioned are listed at the end of the book. The content of the book is based heavily on my experience with many children, young adults and families, but I do want to recognize people and programs from whom I have drawn evidence, inspiration or support.

Introduction

To sail one's own S-H-I-P

Parents everywhere want their children, including those on the autism spectrum, to grow up to be able to sail their own ships: to be Safe, Happy, Independent and Productive.

Many factors contribute to a successful adulthood, including natural talents, family support, education and other learned skills, personal effort and opportunities. Any individual's independence and productivity will differ with these and other variables, but ideally everyone should have the opportunity to maximize his or her own potential.

One very important skill needed throughout life is communication. It is also one of the key areas of difficulty for people on the autism spectrum. In fact, absent, limited or atypical speech and language often lead parents to seek help for their child even before an autism diagnosis is considered.

Communication affects safety, happiness, independence and productivity across domains. For example, if Jake learns to ask for a drink with words, signs or picture symbols instead of hitting or screaming, and Sarah learns to answer questions instead of echoing them, and Derek learns to express his opinion without using rude words and tone, they will have improved their cognition, behavior and social skills as well as their communication.

The purpose of this book

This book will help speech/language pathologists, teachers and parents of autistic children to teach functional communication skills which are developmentally attainable, immediately practical and of lifelong usefulness to the child and future adult. I will provide 11 chapters of consultation to maximize this progress.

Instead of focusing on diagnosis or new breakthroughs or particular treatment programs, this book is about common issues faced by professionals and families working with children who have different levels of development and varied degrees of autism severity. Mostly, it is about ways to move forward.

I believe we can maximize adult potential by individualizing childhood goals and therapies so that the skills addressed will be attainable, useful immediately and a solid basis for future progress for the child in front of you. Your son, daughter or student will be an autistic child for about 20 years but may then be an autistic adult for 60 years or more. It is essential to select and work on skills that will be important now *and* in the future.

In this book, I present nine children and teens, divided into three groups based on their communication development. These will include nonverbal children, those with moderately functional speech or atypical language such as echolalia, and the highly verbal individuals who until recently have been diagnosed with Asperger syndrome.

This book will focus mainly on specific ways to improve communication abilities for the children in these subgroups. Since communication does not occur in a vacuum, the selected goals will also impact behavior and social interaction.

Experience and evidence

I have been fascinated with, and marinating in, the field of autism for more than 40 years, through my career as a speech/language pathologist and autism consultant. I have known many dozens of individuals on the autism spectrum, and usually their families, while working in residential settings, schools and preschools, hospitals, a university and private practice. Often, these relationships have spanned 20 years or more. I have done a lot of speech and language evaluations and therapy, but the majority of my career has been as a consultant to many different public school teams and families working with children and young adults on the autism spectrum for the purpose of increasing communication, independence and appropriate behavior. I have done autism presentations at conferences, in-service events and short courses, distributed e-newsletters to professional colleagues and contributed articles to *Autism Parenting Magazine*.

This book is a compilation of some of the things I have learned along the way from the wonderful children and families I have been privileged to know. My experience includes children and youth of all ages and abilities, many of whom have shared their lives with me over several years or though their entire school years and into adulthood. The recommended goals and detailed teaching methods in this book are designed for speech/language pathologists and teachers to use in schools or clinics, for parents to use at home and for teams to consider in program planning.

My approach to intervention is rooted in the field of communication disorders with strong developmental and behaviorist influences. I value and draw inspiration and support from the research evidence and experiences of all these fields.

The American Speech-Language-Hearing Association (ASHA) is the national organization of speech/language pathologists and audiologists. In a position statement by the Joint Coordinating Committee on Evidence-Based Practice, ASHA describes evidence-based practice as "an approach in which current, high-quality research evidence is integrated with practitioner expertise and client preferences and values into the process of making clinical decisions" (ASHA 2005, p.1).

An extensive review by Wong *et al.* (2014) lists more than 20 therapeutic approaches that have sufficient research support to be considered evidence-based. These include approaches thickly woven through my intervention procedures in the chapters of this book such as:

- modeling
- prompting
- naturalistic intervention
- reinforcement
- scripts
- social narratives
- functional communication training
- visual supports
- Picture Exchange Communication System (PECS).

You will also find threads of my philosophy in statements like:

- Autism is nobody's fault.
- Most children, families and teachers are doing the best they can with what they know right now.
- A team of family and professionals working together can be the child's greatest asset.
- Despite diagnostic similarities, autistic people are individuals first.
- What we choose to teach, and may spend many hours teaching, must meet the child's ability level and be useful in his life, now and in the future.
- Some skills can be readily taught and practiced in a natural environment, and others maybe more efficiently introduced in a

structured setting, but none are truly mastered and useful until they are generalized to real-life situations.

• A lot of behavioral issues result from anxiety and a mismatch between ability and expectations.

• Intensive intervention and tangible reinforcers are often needed to motivate children to change.

Professionals and parents who have written references about my consultation have described me as having a "wealth of knowledge, experience and wisdom," as being "realistic, respectful and encouraging" and "a steadying influence on sometimes contentious teams," with consultation reports that are "concise and timely" and that offer "practical suggestions for intervention" which are "sensible, doable and effective." I appreciate their affirming words and try to live up to them.

The flow of the book

The body of the book is divided into three parts, with each part made up of three chapters dedicated to one of the three communication groups:

Part I: Children with little or no means of expressive communication.

Part II: Children with echolalia or moderately functional speech.

Part III: Children with advanced language skills but poor social communication.

The first two chapters in each part will describe the communicative strengths and concerns of children in that group, and will explain the skills, needs and behaviors of three children or teens. Three or more communication goals will be written for each child and followed with specific descriptions of how to meet the goals.

The third chapter in each part will consider that communication group in more depth, including other relevant skills to teach and further information about important teaching methods. I will also comment on behavior concerns, data keeping, generalization of learned skills and ideas for adults.

The final chapter of the book will consider how some of the frequently recommended methods and supportive techniques were used to improve communication and behavior among children with differing abilities along the spectrum. There will be mention of the evidence base for these methods and of other professionals who developed or use similar practices. Comments from adults on the autism spectrum and professionals who work with them illustrate the need to consider the impact of anxiety when helping autistic children become more comfortable, cooperative and communicative.

Chapter 1

The People in this Book

The children in this book all have a diagnosis of autism spectrum disorder (ASD). Autism is called a spectrum disorder because it includes a wide range of abilities and difficulties. Of course, despite the range of differences, there are similarities required for diagnosis on the autism spectrum.

Three levels of severity on the autism spectrum are included in the diagnosis based on the amount of support the individual needs in life. Specific current diagnostic and severity criteria for ASD can be found in the fifth edition of the American Psychiatric Association's, *Diagnostic and Statistical Manual of Mental Disorders (DSM-5)* (APA 2013, pp.50–59). The diagnostic criteria are paraphrased here.

The differences associated with autism, often called deficits, include social communication and interpersonal interaction that are significantly atypical and occur in many life situations, in comparison with other children of the same age and intellectual development. Those on the autism spectrum have difficulty using and understanding the nonverbal communication that occurs through eye gaze, gestures and facial expression, as well as significant limitations in playing imaginatively, developing friendships and adapting their behavior to different situations (APA 2013, pp.50–51).

Some of them do these things

Daisy does not respond to greetings, and her siblings can't coax her to play with them. Dustin will play-act a movie script, but shrieks if the other children don't know all the lines as he does. Jess flips the table over if she loses a game, and she won't eat meals with her family. Erica blurts out her ideas while others are talking, corrects her teacher and thinks it is a compliment when a classmate rolls his eyes and says, "Sorry we aren't all as smart as you!" Mark spends all his waking hours at home cloistered in his room reading graphic novels or gaming on his computer, and he tries hard to do the same during high school classes and at lunch.

An autism diagnosis also requires some of the following patterns of repetitive behavior, with a limited range of interests and activities (APA 2013, p.50):

- repetitious, non-meaningful actions, use of objects or speech

- rigid insistence on keeping things the same; difficulty shifting from one activity to another

- intense, often unusual interests or attachment to specific objects

- too much or too little reaction to sensory input such as sounds, sights, smells, textures, pain or temperature.

It might look like this

Justin hops and flaps his hands a lot and lines up his cars but does not play with them, Sahara echoes the teacher who is trying to read a story and Seth chants "Bitty bitty bee, bitty bee, bitty bee" repeatedly. Louis will not enter his house without touching a specific tree first, Ben will only eat fish sticks if given three on his plate and Amy won't get out of the car if her mother drives to school by a different route. Joe screams and throws himself on the floor if parted from his plastic shark, Mike asks everyone he sees their birth date and license plate number and

Steven lectures casual acquaintances on the topic of subatomic particles. Jarrett cannot tolerate being in the boys' bathroom at school with other children because of the reverberating noise, but he loves to go in there all alone and make noises he can control. Katie is very upset if someone touches her, but Jason, if allowed, would climb inside anyone's clothing to cuddle and would wander outdoors in his pajamas in a snowstorm.

For a diagnosis to be made, the symptoms of autism must have been present in early childhood, even if they are not recognized until social expectations increase or even if spectrum symptoms have become less obvious because new skills have been learned. To warrant a diagnosis, the differences must truly interfere with important aspects of the person's life. If intellectual disability is present, as is often the case, the autism characteristics must be significant in relation to the person's level of intellectual development rather than his age (APA 2013, pp.50–51).

Although their development is often delayed in relation to their age peers, autistic children are not just behind their peers on the path but are traveling on a different route.

This book's grouping based on communication ability

In my experience, children on the autism spectrum who are at similar developmental levels share some communicative strengths and weaknesses. Despite individual differences, they often benefit from similar goals and teaching procedures. Therefore, the children described in this book are divided into three approximate groups based on their communication profiles and cognitive characteristics and needs. The goals and procedures described here came up frequently in my career and should be applicable to quite a few children on the autism spectrum.

But it is important to remember that the child or children who inspired you to read this book may not rest neatly in one group but may straddle the border between two groups or may grow from one group into the next. Goals and teaching methods recommended for children at the borders of these groups will often be applicable to a child in the adjacent group.

The diagnostic features of autism and other commonalities will show up in a variety of children, but everyone is still an individual first. That said, here are the three groupings created for this book.

The *pre-symbolic communication and emerging speech* group includes children, teens and even adults who are nonverbal or say only a few words and don't have a strong alternative means of communication such as American Sign Language (ASL), picture exchange or a speech-generating device (SGD). That is, they have little or no use of spoken or visible symbols to express meaning. They often also have limited understanding of speech, may exhibit behaviors such as wandering, bolting, unsafe climbing, aggression or loud emotional meltdowns, and show little conventional use of toys and objects such as eating utensils, toothbrushes and books. But they may know how to run some of your electronics. This category, like the other two, is based on present level of functioning, not the age of the individual.

The members of the *atypical language* group, which may include some graduates from the pre-symbolic group, may be speaking in many single words and some phrases or in sentences, with varying clarity of speech. Or they may be using long sentences spoken very clearly but obviously echoed from things other people have just said or have said in a similar situation in the past. Echoed sentences may even be spoken by the autistic child in the foreign accent of the original speaker. Memory is strong, but comprehension of other people's language, although better than in the pre-symbolic group, is still an issue. In my experience, echolalia has never been accompanied by solid understanding of the speech of others. Noisy distress, bolting or aggression and perseverative repetition of words and phrases may occur. The child may use functional objects and toys appropriately, such as running a comb through hair or pushing a train on a track, but imaginative play or social play with peers is unlikely to have developed without direct instruction.

In the *advanced language with gaps* group we find those who would previously have been diagnosed with Asperger syndrome. They have much stronger understanding and use of speech and language than the two previous groups, whether they are reticent and withdrawn or extremely (sometimes excessively!) talkative. They would score in the normal or superior range of ability on tests of intellectual capacity, but struggle with understanding non-literal language such as idioms or sarcasm and recognizing the meaning of the nonverbal body language that often supports or negates the intent of natural conversation. They may make comments in words and tone of voice that others hear as rude, and tend to monologue on favorite topics regardless of the listeners' interest. Behavioral outbursts are still common, often in response to anxiety or frustration.

The characteristics of members of these three groups, their significant needs, recommended goals and the specific methods to help them make meaningful progress will be the substance of the coming chapters. My groupings are descriptive, not diagnostic. The purpose of describing the three groups and nine children is to share therapy methods which will be useful for children with similar developmental profiles.

Although the adult outcomes for this wide range of individuals will surely differ from each other, it is possible, and necessary, to guide them toward lives in which they can be safe, feel happiness and contentment, and have some degree of independent functioning. They may become somewhat, or even very, productive, whether this means helping unload the dishwasher in a group home, organizing the produce section in a market or teaching in a university.

What do we mean by sailing one's own S-H-I-P?

The major goal of this book is to help therapists, teachers and parents assist children on the autism spectrum to be the captains of their own lives to the greatest extent possible. None of us learns to sail our personal life ship with safety, happiness, independence and productivity without instruction and help, and autistic individuals especially need to work on this during childhood as well as in adulthood. The S-H-I-P goals as I see them are as follows:

- **Safety:** This could mean anything from not running into traffic to judging when it is safe to pull into the intersection while driving. In communication terms, it might mean being able to say or show where it hurts, to tell a policeman you have autism or to abstain from scolding a motorcycle gang for smoking. The safety of others matters too, so teaching interactive skills, such as effectively communicating a need or anxiety without aggression, are key to protecting others and shielding the person on the autism spectrum from the consequences of using aggressive behaviors.

- **Happiness:** Here, I mean contentment, a minimum of anxiety and comfortable enjoyment of a life of one's choosing. One autistic person may find happiness in the freedom to walk alone along a fenced-in trail and another might experience it through sharing political opinions with a like-minded audience. Quite possibly neither will show enthusiastic verbal or facial expressions of joy or satisfaction.

- **Independence:** Of course, levels of independence will vary greatly with the individual's cognitive, physical, verbal and social abilities, but the goal is to maximize everyone's degree of control over his or her own life. Being able to express one's preferences, choose to interact or withdraw at times and accomplish daily living activities with little or no help may be some of the most basic aspects of independence. For those at more advanced levels of achievement, the goal might be living and working independently, being a spouse or parent, and moving beyond independence to dependability and interdependence.

- **Productivity:** We all have different talents, weaknesses and motivations, but if we are contributing to others, we are being productive. Some people known or presumed to have autism, including some who are otherwise very dependent, have made significant and creative contributions in art, music, science and literature. However, the person who has learned to dress himself, help re-shelve the library books or tutor middle school students in math is also being productive.

How do we help?

My philosophy is that autism is nobody's fault, that most autistic people and their caregivers are doing the best they can at the moment, and that a team working together can accomplish a lot more than the same people working individually. The core of the team is the child, surrounded by his parents and other family members, all being assisted by any or all of these people: speech/language pathologists (SLPs), occupational therapists (OTs), physical therapists (PTs), teachers and paraprofessionals, Applied Behavior Analysis (ABA) specialists, principals and special education administrators, psychologists, doctors, psychiatrists, guidance counselors and social workers, music and art therapists, dietitians, and others.

What does the team need to do?

- Most of all, work together. A coordinated, cooperating team can be the child's greatest educational asset.

- Remember that other team members will come and go in the life of the growing child, but the family will remain and must be an integral part of the process. In my experience, programs that include parents as part of the teaching team have generally seen greater and longer-lasting progress than those that do not.

- Develop a plan that is realistic, optimistic and flexible, and recognizes the challenges the child faces, the progress that has been made and the obstacles that arise. And be ready to adjust the teaching process accordingly as you work diligently to implement the plan. Aim high, in small steps.

- Establish goals that are practical, developmentally appropriate and useful for increasing independence, both now and in the future.

- Be sure the team members know each other's goals, have strategies for incorporating them through the day and stay in frequent contact about glitches and progress. Expect your work to be a collaborative challenge.

- Support the family and help them develop the grit to keep going when their nonverbal twin toddlers are biting them and escaping from their bedroom windows onto the porch roof, when their child will only eat a few white- and tan-colored foods, when their teen withdraws to his room and computer most of his waking hours, or when their college-educated young adult refuses to apply for 80% of available jobs because of uncompromising moral beliefs, unrealistically high or low self-assessment of abilities, feelings of entitlement, or anxiety or sensory concerns.

- But also savor the joys with them: when those toddlers learn to use words or signs or pictures to make requests, when three new foods become acceptable to the child, when the teen tells his mother "I love you" for the first time and the young adult gets a part-time job.

Now that everyone is working together, what about those goals?

School systems and early childhood programs have established ways that they believe goals and objectives must be written and measured. However, these are not the same everywhere and they are revised from time to time, so for the purposes of this book, we will use the term "goals" for both long- and short-term plans. Determining how long it should take, how to measure progress and what levels of performance indicate that a goal is mastered are also important, but our major focus will be on choosing and accomplishing goals that enhance communication, safety, happiness, independence and productivity.

Although the people in this book have invented names and the characteristics of more than one real individual, the events, procedures and progress are real and have occurred multiple times in my career.

As a team considers language-related goals for each of these three communication subgroups of the autism spectrum, it is important to ask:

Is the goal developmentally appropriate?

Is this child ready to learn this skill? This is a key measure of whether it is attainable. The expectation should exceed the child's present level of ability, but not too greatly. Setting lofty goals of what we would like to see happen might feel good at the planning meeting, but if they are too far beyond the child's ability, they are much less likely to be met and may mean that earlier steps which could have been accomplished are not attempted.

Is it functional?

Will it be useful? Does accomplishment of this goal really help the learner live a safer, happier, more independent and/or more productive life? Not every objective will meet all these criteria, but each one should further some of these goals.

Will it provide a platform for future progress?

For example, learning to wait is a step toward being able to survive a trip to a restaurant or store, accurately answering "Yes" or "No" helps a child express preferences and demonstrate knowledge, and learning to negotiate politely will be vital in employment.

Can the team provide the program?

Do we have the time, people and other resources needed to help the child reach this goal, and if not, how can we get them?

Do we need to make a change?

If the child in your communication program is making good progress and has goals that are functional, developmentally appropriate and useful now and in the future, then, no. If together you are struggling, try the ideas in this book.

How do we do it?

This book will help answer that question for a variety of important communication goals. The coming chapters will introduce some children at different levels of communication development, describe their past learning and present needs, and provide some appropriate goals and specific ways to meet them. These particular needs and goals are not often seen in typical or delayed speech and language development, but they reflect common language and behavior differences of ASD.

PART I

PRE-SYMBOLIC COMMUNICATION AND EMERGING SPEECH

Chapter 2

Communicating
Without Speech

Rebecca

Words, spoken or written, are symbols. They reliably represent, or stand for, something real, such as an object, action or concept. Photos, drawings and the signs of American Sign Language (ASL) are also symbols that have consistent recognizable meaning. Speech is the oral, out loud, expression of language symbols. Autistic people who are in the pre-symbolic group have not yet learned to use symbols to express themselves and probably also have severe limitations in understanding the symbols used by others. That is, typically both their expressive (spoken, signed, picture-based, written) language and their receptive (heard, seen or read, understood) language are significantly impaired. With autism, this severe language deficit is often accompanied by significant disability in cognitive and adaptive living skills such as using toys appropriately or eating, toileting and dressing independently.

Pre-symbolic children on the autism spectrum rarely compensate for their lack of symbolic language by using gestures, facial expression or consistent vocal sounds to convey their desires and intentions clearly. The early communication of autistic children has often included taking an adult's hand and putting it on or near a desired item. This is apt to be done by the child without looking at the adult's face. It appears as if the child is using the adult's hand as a tool, and it does not involve use of symbols, but it does signal intent to accomplish something.

In contrast, a typically developing young toddler, or a pre-verbal child who is deaf or has a severe motor speech disorder, but not autism, is likely to find more varied ways to signal meaning. For example, those children might reach for or point to a cup of juice on the table while making a vocal noise to get your attention and looking back and forth between you and the cup. In the same situation, the pre-symbolic child with autism may stand by the table looking at the juice and screaming or whining without actively involving you.

Children typically show a variety of communicative functions before learning to talk. These include waving, pointing and looking where you point or look, clapping, smiling and looking at you to show pleasure, shaking their heads to refuse or protest, or looking to a parent when frightened. These communicative behaviors are frequently absent or occur rarely among pre-symbolic children on the autism spectrum.

Without intervention, these children's behaviors are often solitary, even if they are twins, and may not seem purposeful. Examples include flicking ribbons or strings, picking up and dropping toys, spinning objects, opening and closing doors, or flushing and watching the toilet water over and over. Many are attracted to electronic screens and may re-watch the same videos many times, often becoming skilled at repeatedly replaying favorite parts. There may be repetitive vocal noises, lack of response to verbal directions, resistance to being physically assisted or directed, and loud noisy distress, and perhaps aggression, if the child is thwarted, pressured or over-stimulated.

Are they stuck there?

It depends. Some young children with these characteristics progress to develop emerging or even moderately good language. Others unfortunately remain nonverbal and pre-symbolic through adulthood. Regardless of the eventual outcome, there is room for growth and im-provement in communication and independence at all ages and stages of development. And each step of that growth can enhance the individual's quality of life.

Let's meet a few children, here and in future chapters, and see how they progress. The children I describe have assumed names but share the characteristics of many real children I have known. They will be introduced with brief descriptions of their characteristics and relevant aspects of their histories. Then the major focus will be on appropriate functional goals and descriptions of ways to meet those goals.

Rebecca

Rebecca is an 11-year-old girl who is nonverbal and has limited understanding of spoken language. She does occasionally appear to understand some frequently used sentences such as "Let's go for a ride" or "It's time for lunch," but she does not respond to them reliably. When she does respond, it may be because of additional cues, such as seeing classmates lining up at the door.

In addition to special education, occupational therapy and physical therapy, Rebecca has had years of speech/language therapy, with an emphasis initially on speech and then on alternative/augmentative communication (AAC) including American Sign Language (ASL) and use of picture communication in a speech-generating device (SGD) and through picture exchange with no technology. Language comprehension and speech did not develop, the motor and conceptual aspects of manual signs proved too difficult, and Rebecca did not appear to recognize that pictures represented real objects. At age nine, she was introduced to an object choice system for requesting free-time activities and an object-based schedule for school activities.

Choices

A major first goal was to help Rebecca indicate some of her desires. Since she did not recognize pictures as symbols of real foods or toys, her team developed a choice board using small objects as symbols, in the hope that these would be realistic enough to be meaningful to Rebecca.

Her choice board is a piece of plywood the size of a large pizza, painted green and screwed into the concrete block wall of her classroom. Spots of Velcro™ allow the choice symbols to be arrayed in random positions on the green circle board. The symbols, partially embedded in squares of tri-wall cardboard, are small objects such as a piece of a pool noodle, a few large beads or a Duplo™ block to represent some of her free-time toy choices.

Initially, Rebecca was shown the choice board with only a single symbol on it, such as the symbol for the beads. She was assisted to pull the symbol off and hand it to her teacher, and then she immediately received her bead toy. She began to learn that giving someone a symbol was a request. This first symbol was chosen to represent something that Rebecca really wanted—her bead toy.

Then she learned to discriminate between the bead symbol and a blank card, which deliberately represented "nothing." The purpose of the blank card was to teach her to pause, look and think before pulling off a symbol to make a request. When she gave the blank card to her teacher, the teacher simply said "Blank" and put it back on the board.

At first, Rebecca learned something we didn't mean to teach. She would remove the blank, replace it on the board as her teacher had done, and then pull off her choice symbol and give it to her teacher, apparently believing that this extra step was now necessary. We had to temporarily move the blank to a greater distance from the symbol so she could not easily reach it and then gradually move it closer while guiding her to use only the choice symbol. After she learned to ignore the useless blank and select the bead symbol, other positive choice symbols were added to her board.

We also added a symbol for a negative choice—a hairbrush, because Rebecca hated to have her hair brushed. If she gave her teacher the hairbrush symbol, the teacher would briefly brush Rebecca's hair and replace the symbol on the board. Eventually, she learned to avoid the hairbrush symbol, which was what we hoped would happen. In the meantime, she became more tolerant of having her hair brushed, which was a fortuitous bonus.

By the end of the school year, Rebecca had seven free-time options, any five of which might be available on the choice circle at one time. We test her knowledge of the symbols in two ways. If she selects a symbol and then is offered that toy and another toy, she will take the one she requested 80% of the time, showing that she knows what the different symbols represent.

Likewise, if she is offered two actual toys, Rebecca will reach for one. When her teacher pulls back the toys and moves her own hand near the choice board, Rebecca will select the symbol that matches the toy she reached for 80% of the time and put the symbol in her teacher's hand. She will play with the chosen item for 5–10 minutes, giving it back when a timer beeps.

A schedule

Rebecca's daily schedule at school rotates among table-work times, walks and gym times, bathroom trips, snacks and lunch, and free-time choices. Transitioning between any two of these activities was distressing to Rebecca and, therefore, painful for the teachers she hit or kicked during transitions. Since picture schedules had been unsuccessful, an object symbol schedule was created.

Rebecca's schedule is a strip of wall paneling 18 inches long and seven inches wide. Symbols are arranged in a left-to-right sequence on the schedule strip, and each is removed after the activity it represents is finished. A green plastic circle symbol on her schedule indicates that it is time for her to choose a free-time activity from the wall-mounted choice board. A doll-house toilet indicates bathroom time, a faux wood countertop sample means it is time for table work, and a miniature sneaker represents a walk.

The schedule strip was introduced by just adding it to her expected routine with a simple script in which her teacher would say "Time for table work," tap that symbol and immediately present a task. When the activity was done, she would say "Table work is done," remove the symbol from the schedule and drop it in a "finished" box. She would then tap the next symbol, saying "Time for free choice," and guide Rebecca to her choice board on the wall.

Initially, Rebecca appeared to ignore her teacher's recitations of the schedule, but gradually she began to watch and then to help move the completed symbols to the finished box. Later, she started to recognize the meaning of the symbols and would sometimes go to the next scheduled location as her teacher removed the symbol for the just-completed activity.

It is important to note that without the symbols Rebecca did not, and still does not, reliably understand even routine spoken instructions. For example, if she finishes her table-work session and her teacher says "Time for snack," but does not show her the snack symbol, Rebecca will not move from her seat. However, as soon as the snack symbol is placed on her schedule she will hop up and go to the kitchen area. Rebecca has demonstrated this dependence on the visual symbols consistently, and it is a good illustration of how vital this visual support is to her functional communication.

Initially, she was resistant to instructional work at a table, which included basic matching and sorting tasks and puzzle assembly, but with reinforcement from small treats and use of the schedule, Rebecca has become more cooperative and less inclined to whack or kick adults who approach her with expectations. Now, she reliably goes to her table when shown the table-work symbol on her schedule, and sometimes she just goes there between activities to wait for her next instructions. Her school day runs more smoothly, and she appears relaxed and content most of the time.

Since she occasionally balks about returning from a walk, her adult helper carries the green circle symbol in a pocket and shows it to Rebecca before she begins to resist, saying "Time for free choice," and Rebecca will usually head back to her classroom and go directly to the choice board. Not all of her free-time choices are on the circle board all the time, and on occasion Rebecca has looked at the board, then turned to the storage box of other choice symbols on a nearby shelf, selected one of those and handed it to the adult working with her. We were pleased to see her find a creative way to tell us that we were not offering what she wanted.

With the use of object symbols, Rebecca has gradually developed good ability to choose a desired activity and to understand and follow a familiar routine calmly. Expressing preferences is a major step in independence, as is her emerging ability to predict and initiate a next step in her schedule. Decreased aggression makes everyone safer, Rebecca is more content and productive at school, and similar systems have been set up at home.

What communication goals should we target next?

Rebecca's program could be, and will be, expanded to increase the number and type of choices available to her and the variety of activities on her schedule, and to gradually decrease the amount of help she requires on table work and self-help tasks. But another change, which will require, and develop, cognitive growth, is also planned.

The team, while pleased with Rebecca's progress, would like her to have a less cumbersome, more conventional and perhaps more portable style of visual schedule and choices, so the plan is to gradually shift from three-dimensional objects to two-dimensional picture symbols in her schedule and choice board. The team's hope is that she might eventually use a basic speech-generating device (SGD) that will speak her choices aloud, in addition to her present non-technological systems. Here are some new goals for Rebecca:

Goal #1: Rebecca will maintain her current level of accuracy when using pictures instead of objects to represent her present vocabulary of choice and schedule items.

Remember that Rebecca has already shown difficulty understanding that pictures can represent real objects. You should expect the shift to two-dimensional symbols to require a series of steps.

First, take photos of the object symbols she is using now, not pictures of the toys themselves or Rebecca using the toys, but close-up photos of the actual symbols she has been giving you to make requests and has seen on her schedule.

Attach these photos to her object symbols so that she sees both the object and the picture together, and print the name of the item or activity under the picture so all adults will call it by the same name. When possible, choose names that will be age-appropriate as she grows, such as "bathroom" or "toilet" instead of "potty."

When these two-part symbols are familiar to Rebecca, select one of her favorite choice items and cut off the object half so that symbol on her circular choice board is now only a picture. But do not discard the object symbols. If she is still able to use the picture-only symbol effectively, gradually do the same with other symbols until you have eventually removed all the object symbols. You may still need to start with object symbols when introducing new vocabulary. If she is not able to make the shift to picture symbols, or can do so with some symbols and not others, go back to the object symbols as needed.

As was done with the object system, use few spoken words and phrases during schedule and choice activities. If Rebecca gives you the bead symbol, just say "Beads!" as you take the symbol and "Beads!" again as you give her the bead toy. This frequent, uncomplicated repetition will make it more likely that she will learn to understand the name of the item than if you embed the key words in a sentence like "Oh, I see you want..." or "Okay, here are your..."

For some parts of the schedule, you may speed the recognition of the picture symbols if you have her carry the object-plus-picture symbol to the location of the activity it represents and match it to a picture-only symbol there. For example, she might carry the two-part symbol of the toilet or her worktable and place it on a matching picture symbol laminated onto a bathroom table or her work surface. This can also serve to remind her where she is going and as a hall pass facsimile. It supports her understanding of the important distinction that if she gives you a symbol, she is asking for something, and if you give her one, she is expected to do something. When traveling between locations, let her lead the way whenever possible.

As you shift her materials to less cumbersome two-dimensional ones, keep the choice items arranged randomly on a circular display and keep the schedule linear. The schedule could be set up as a top-to-bottom "list," but since Rebecca is accustomed to a left-to-right schedule arrangement, it would be wise to maintain that for her. These two styles of symbol arrangement will help illustrate the distinction that schedules get followed in a set order but choices can be selected by preference.

Goal #2: When noticing a person holding or eating something she wants, Rebecca will approach the person and extend her hand, palm up, as a request to use or share the desired item.

Rebecca already has some skills related to this goal. If an adult is nearby, she will hold out her cup to indicate that she wants more to drink. She sometimes signs a fair approximation of "more" as a general "I want" request for something she sees someone else eating. Other times she just grabs it.

To help her learn to request to use or share something she sees someone else using or eating, set up temptations such as an adult eating popcorn nearby. If she shows interest, help her to approach that person and extend her hand, palm up. The adult with the popcorn can say "Popcorn!" and give her a few pieces, then move to another location so Rebecca can practice approaching and asking again. The adult assisting Rebecca should say nothing; this is supposed to be an interaction between Rebecca and the person with the popcorn. The extra adult should just silently assist and gradually withdraw the non-verbal prompts as Rebecca becomes more independent. If she learns this easily, you could add having her sign "please" as she asks. This is a relatively easy sign to do (place palm flat on chest and move your hand in a circular motion) because it uses only one hand, requires no finger positioning and makes contact with the body. It is easier to do than "I want" and is a nice suggestion of politeness.

Goal #3: Rebecca will complete three different problem-solving activities without assistance.

This goal builds on the six different table-work activities that Rebecca has been doing with her teacher. She now requires help from her teacher with all these activities, so we chose three of them for her to learn to do independently. We want Rebecca to be able to be productive even when an adult is not right with her, to direct herself instead of waiting for direction in a familiar situation, to maintain her focus through a short task and to self-correct when she encounters small glitches.

This is a precursor to the independent work described in the third goal for Seth in Chapter 6. After they have learned to do a variety of activities to completion by themselves, many pre-symbolic children can also complete a sequence of independent work happily and successfully.

The three activities for Rebecca will be a box with a slot and eight large plastic "coins" to drop in the slot, a four-piece puzzle of basic shapes with knobs to hold on to, and a small pegboard with ten pegs. The materials were chosen with Rebecca's strengths and weaknesses in mind. She enjoys putting things into slots and holes. But because she has limited dexterity, the "coins" are thick enough for her to pick up easily, the puzzle pieces have knobs and will not fit into the wrong holes, and the pegs are chunky and widely spaced in the pegboard. For now, these will all be separate tasks. Rebecca will not be expected to transition from one to the next by herself, as she would in the independent work sequence described in Chapter 6.

Rebecca has been working on these tasks for a couple of months, but she will still need teacher assistance for a while. The puzzle will be the most difficult for Rebecca because it is more cognitively and motorically challenging. Some ways to decrease her dependence on teacher assistance include:

- Be as unobtrusive as possible. Resist the urge to help if she is trying to figure out something on her own. And be quiet. Her comprehension of language is very poor, and she won't be helped by verbal instructions.

- Put the loose pieces (coins, shapes and pegs) in a basket beside the box or board they will go into. That way, they won't be dropping on the floor and she can easily see when the task is done.

- Give as much help as necessary but as little as possible. Prompt her gently, minimally and nonverbally. If she is gazing into space, try to just nudge her elbow so she reaches toward the pegs instead of putting a peg in her hand. If she is struggling to put the square in the puzzle and seems about to give up, push the edge of the square toward the hole instead of helping hand over hand.

- You may need to put away the pegboard and puzzle as soon as she is finished or Rebecca may start taking pieces out, which negates the idea of completing a task.

- A small treat at the end may help her recognize and aim for completion sooner. Rebecca is partial to cheese balls.

Some other communication skills that would be helpful for Rebecca include learning to "wait" and developing some visually supported understanding of the names of common objects. These will be addressed in Arnie's program in the next chapter, but, now or later, may be applicable to Rebecca as well.

Chapter 3

Early Language Comprehension and Expression

Arnie and Darius

Communication is bigger than speech. Much significant information has been conveyed and many valuable relationships have developed through writing, sign language and voice output communication devices. Just consider Helen Keller and Stephen Hawking. But speech is everywhere, and highly desired. Working on alternative means of communication does not mean giving up on helping children understand and use speech.

The two boys in this chapter are younger than Rebecca and have somewhat more advanced abilities in cognition and communication, but they are still essentially pre-symbolic. The goals for Arnie will target language comprehension, and those for Darius will focus on spoken language and play. These are important goals, but not their whole communication program. Both boys will continue to use picture communication to support their receptive and expressive language development.

Arnie

Arnie is seven and has learned to exchange a few pictures to make requests. He will spontaneously remove a ketchup symbol that is Velcroed onto the table near his seat and give it to his mother at mealtimes. Arnie eats ketchup on everything. He also has two separate choice boards, one with three options for toys and the other with symbols for sensory choices such as a weighted blanket, a stretchy tunnel and a small trampoline. He does not reliably seek these choice boards but will make a selection if his parents give him the choice boards, and the sensory choices often calm him if offered before he is extremely distressed. He also pulls his mother or father to the refrigerator, cupboard or front door (all of which have childproof locks) and puts the parent's hand on the door handles to indicate that he wants something to eat or to go out.

He feeds himself with his fingers, and sometimes a spoon and cup, is not toilet trained, and often wanders in the house at night. He does not recognize boundaries or safety concerns, and may dash off in dangerous situations if his hand is not tightly held. He does not reliably stop or come if called and is sometimes resistant or aggressive if moved against his wishes. When engaged in teaching activities, Arnie may giggle perseveratively, or bite and scratch at apparently random, but frequent, times.

Clearly, Arnie has educational needs in many life skills areas, including expressive communication, and the team will address these, but here we will focus on his receptive language—his understanding of the words he hears. These goals might also be appropriate for Rebecca.

Goal #1: Arnie will reliably comply with instructions to "Give me" an object in his hand, and to "Come here" from a distance of 12 feet.

This goal is going to require some strong positive reinforcement and probably physical prompting at first, but the goal won't be met until he can do these things without a physical prompt. The reinforcer, or reward given to increase the likelihood that he will respond the same way next time, needs to be given immediately after his response. It should be given very often at first and must be something he really wants. A small food treat, sometimes as small as half a chocolate-covered raisin or a piece of diced apple, usually works best, though for Arnie it may have to be something dipped in ketchup. He really wants the tangle of strings he likes to flick in front of his eyes, but since you don't want to keep taking it away from him so you can continue practicing, a consumable will probably be better. You might give him the strings at longer pauses as you rearrange teaching materials.

"Give me"

For "Give me," put one or more common objects on a table in front of him, and after Arnie has picked one up and perhaps looked at it a little, hold out your hand, palm up and say "Give me" and the name of the object ("Give me the comb"). Be sure to use items that will be in his life forever so that their names are worth knowing. Several things could happen here, not counting Arnie bolting from the table, and you will respond accordingly.

He gives you the item. You say "Comb!" and give him the treat. Have it ready in your other hand and give it to him as you say the name of the item. If you can't easily put it in his hand, just put it on the table in front of him. It is important that he receives it immediately after giving you the requested object.

He waves the item by his face and does not appear to notice that you have spoken to him. You move his hand to your hand, take the comb and finish as if he had given it to you himself, saying "Comb!" and delivering the treat. It is even better if a second adult, or a sibling perhaps, sits beside or behind him and moves his arm. That person should not speak. All we want Arnie to hear is the name of the item and the instruction "Give me." The silent assistant should help as little as possible and gradually decrease the prompting as Arnie begins to respond more readily.

He doesn't pick up one of the items. Then you or your helper assist him to do so. Also, practice "Give me" in more natural settings when he does already happen to have something in his hand, being sure to name it enthusiastically and give the treat when you have the requested object in your hand. Be sure you have the reinforcer in your hand before you make the request. Remember, during the table task he doesn't have to find the object you name; you name the one he is holding.

He gives it to you and then holds his hand out, palm up. You could give it back to him, naming it cheerfully as you do so if you think that is what he wants. However, if he's been doing this activity for a while, it is more likely that he is asking for the reinforcer, so I would give him that.

"Come here"

To teach "Come here," start with him sitting in a chair a few feet from you and call "Arnie, come here," and use a beckoning hand gesture. Have a silent assistant nudge him to you and you reward him with a treat. You can add verbal praise, and a hug or pat if he enjoys these. Skip the physical contact during this practice if it is not rewarding or is upsetting to Arnie. Otherwise, you may teach him to avoid coming! Gradually increase the distance between you and be sure to practice, with the reward, in natural situations also.

> **Goal #2**: Arnie will "wait" when requested for up to 20 seconds, with visual cues but no physical prompting.

Learning to "wait" is also a skill that typically requires patient teaching for pre-symbolic students, but it returns good value. It can significantly impact safety concerns. One could even say the child who can wait is being "productive" if the alternative is bolting and needing to be chased.

To teach the action of waiting to children or adults who have no reliable understanding of the word or concept, I have used the following procedure, adapted from the Picture Exchange Communication System (Frost and Bondy 2002, pp.258–261).

Create a visible symbol that is unlike other pictures/symbols that Arnie is using for communication. It should be bigger, sturdy, colorful and appealing to hold. I like rubber jar openers or similar circles or ovals of stretchy or textured pliable rubber, but a laminated piece of poster board will do. Since Arnie may decide to fling it, something soft is best. I write "WAIT" on it, mostly so the adults remember what it is for. It's good to have several, as you may want one in the car, bathroom or pocket of an accompanying caregiver.

Practice at first with Arnie seated at a table or desk. When he finishes a table task, remove the task materials, give him the WAIT symbol, and say and sign "Wait" (hold both hands up and off to the side a bit, fingers pointing up, palms toward you; wiggle the fingers). Pairing the symbol with the word and sign increases the possibility that eventually the word or sign will be sufficient without the symbol.

Quickly (for some children this must be *very* quickly at first), but smoothly, produce a reinforcer (a consumable treat usually works well) and trade it for the symbol, as you say something like "Waiting's all done," "Good waiting" or "Thanks for waiting." If there will be a pause in the teaching session, this is a good time to use Arnie's strings as the reinforcer.

Ideally, Arnie will be holding the symbol and will hand it back to you, but if not, just take it from the table the first few times. Then, when you've demonstrated several times and have his attention, either prompt him to hold and give back the symbol or, preferably, have another adult silently prompt that behavior from behind. The prompter should be encouraged not to talk, as this typically causes confusion.

Gradually increase the time of the wait—up to 20 seconds for the current goal—and increase the distance between you. That is, give the wait instruction, walk away, delay and come back with the reinforcer.

When Arnie can stay in his seat while you go away, delay and return with the reinforcer, start working with him standing and in different situations. As an example, after he has made a choice or request you might give him the WAIT symbol and delay your response to his request. Then transfer use of the WAIT symbol to less predictable situations, such as when you pause to talk with someone or he must wait with you in a short line.

Expect that this will take considerable practice, especially when you move beyond the table sessions, or only say and/or sign "wait" without giving him the symbol, but it is a very functional lifelong skill that can eventually be useful in many settings.

Another language comprehension goal for Arnie, this one focused on visually supported receptive vocabulary, could be:

Goal #3: Arnie will reliably give an adult any of ten common objects, selected from an array of four, in response to the verbal instruction "Give me the...(name of object)."

This means that you will choose a target vocabulary of ten items with names that are important for him to know, such as spoon, sock, ball, cup and toothbrush, and, after practice, if you put any four of them in front of Arnie, he will be able to give you the one you ask for. This is a more advanced version of the "Give me" section of Goal #1, where you named the item for him and he only needed to understand the "Give me" part.

The problem is that Arnie has been working on this for several months and does not seem to be learning the names of the objects. He will give you something, but it is usually the object closest to him, not necessarily the one you asked for. So let's give him some visual support and create more nearly errorless learning.

Since Arnie clearly does not understand the names of these objects, and that is what we want him to learn, we will add a visual matching component to help him. The purposes are to teach him:

- to understand the names of common objects and

- that the pictures presented to him are instructions to do something.

In all of the following the steps, you say the single-word name of the object or picture every time you touch it or Arnie touches it, and you don't say much else. If you feel sure that some of these numbered steps are too easy, start at a later step and just back up to an earlier level if he is confused.

1. Place a single object (sock) on the table. Hold out your hand, palm up, with an identical sock on the palm of your hand, and say "Sock." Pause... "Give me the sock." If he picks up the one on the table and puts it in your hand (essentially matching it to the sock you are holding), reinforce him with the treat as you say "Sock!" enthusiastically. He has now heard the name of the item three times while seeing and/or touching it. If he does nothing, you or your silent helper can assist him to pick it up and put it in your hand. Reward this just as if he had done it himself. Gradually decrease the help until he is doing it by himself.

2. Repeat #1 with several different objects, having only one object on the table at a time and always showing him an identical matching object. You might practice with a spoon, a comb and a cup, one at a time.

3. When he can reliably give you a single item that matches the one you show him, increase the number of objects on the table so that he has to select the one that you name and show him while he ignores the others. Initially, you may need to make this easier by having the items you didn't ask for a little harder for him to reach.

4. When he can do this with several common objects, change the ones you show him so that they are similar but not identical. For example, you show him a blue sock and the one on the table is white. You still just say "Give me the sock." You may need to temporarily go back to having only the item you ask for on the

table and rebuild up to expecting him to discriminate among several items to find the one you ask for.

5. The next step is to do the same, but now show an identical photo of the object you are requesting. If Arnie can still give you the items you request, you can try showing him just a similar picture, such as a drawing of a sock or comb.

6. Now try doing the activity with no visible sample. Just say the words "Give me the…" with three or four objects on the table. If Arnie can do this, you have some measurable single-word comprehension and can add new words and expand to asking him to retrieve the practiced items in more natural situations. If he still doesn't understand the spoken words, or learns some words and not others, you can use the visual cues as support in natural situations, such as showing him a sock picture and saying "Get your socks."

Other skills to teach

Matching and sorting activities are also good ways to model common vocabulary if you say the target words at carefully planned intervals while Arnie is paying attention to them. For example, help him sort socks from combs as you hand them to him one at a time. Say "Comb" as you give it to him, "Comb" as he moves it toward the comb container, with or without your help, and "Comb!" as he drops it into the container. At random times, after two to four items have been sorted, immediately hand him his reinforcer instead of a sock or comb, naming it "popcorn," "chip" or "raisin" as you give it to him. He will know where to "sort" that one!

Use a similar process for helping him match an object that you give him to a picture on the table, trying to say the vocabulary word three times. Avoid extra language like "No, not there," "Try again" and "Good job" as these are apt to be confusing and take his focus off the vocabulary word you are teaching. Don't keep testing; use errorless learning by helping him match the object to the picture. Gradually decrease your help as he learns to do it himself.

Provide additional vocabulary practice using things that are important to Arnie, such as ketchup, his string tangle or a piece of apple, while teaching him to point specifically to things he wants. Place a favorite item out of reach, direct his attention to it and shape his hand into a pointing gesture. As you help him point to the item, name it two or three times and then give it to him.

Learning to "give" an object he might otherwise have swallowed, to "come" away from the edge of the swimming pool and to "wait" instead of bolting into traffic may keep Arnie safer. He will, of course, still need close supervision. Knowing that things have consistent names and that pictures can support verbal instructions should improve his ability to follow spoken directions and picture schedules with less aberrant behavior. Pointing is a very useful communicative signal for requesting. All of these basic skills help form a platform for further learning.

Darius

Darius is four years old and has learned some early communication skills. He has demonstrated reliable understanding of some short frequently used sentences such as "Time for a bath" and "Do you want a snack?" or "Get your coat." It is likely that he understands these because he knows the key words (bath, snack, coat) and because these short sentences occur in fairly predictable situations. He does not necessarily understand the meaning of each word in the sentences.

Without prompting, he uses a choice board in the kitchen to make requests for different foods. He will take a symbol from the board and give it to one of his parents, even if the parent is in another room. He uses another picture board in the family room to select videos or TV shows. Darius is beginning to try to say some words, especially those that match the symbols on his choice boards, such as "apple," "juice" and "car."

He is an active little boy, often climbing and jumping on furniture, and as a three-year-old he escaped through his bedroom window to the porch roof. He doesn't sit and play with a toy with his parents. His toy use is mainly watching the same videos on a tablet repeatedly, flipping his larger trucks over and spinning their wheels, and lining up his small cars and trucks.

To help Darius learn more efficiently, we need to increase his interaction with, and attention to, a person teaching him, help him begin to use problem-solving toys and encourage imitation of actions and speech.

We could start with three goals. Two of these require directly learning from an adult, but one is more structured and may be easier to accomplish at first, so we'll start there.

Goal #1: Darius will stay seated with an adult and participate in structured joint activities that involve matching, sorting and simple assembly for 20-minute sessions.

To establish an individual teaching routine, choose a workspace that is consistently available, provides stable seating and a flat work surface, and is not easy for Darius to leave spontaneously. Possibilities might include a booster chair at the kitchen table or a small table and chairs with a wall on one side of Darius and you sitting on his other side with your foot hooked around one of his chair legs.

Select activities that are uncomplicated, have a limited number of pieces and involve using his hands. It helps if they can be completed with you helping to move his hands at first if necessary. Choose things that can be done quickly when introduced but can become more challenging as he progresses. Puzzles in which each piece has its own hole, shape sorters and nesting cups are good starter items that involve problem solving and work well with hand-over-hand assistance if Darius needs help or is more inclined to throw them than play with them.

Later, matching and sorting tasks, as described for Arnie, and directed imitation of actions, sounds and words will be good additions, but initially you may need to anchor a puzzle board with one hand, and just help him put in the last, and easiest, piece. Immediately reward this with a treat and a simultaneous social reinforcer like "It's in!" "Yeah!" or "Good!" just as if he had done it by himself. Be sure to have a variety of treats he likes in case he tires of the one you are offering. Sometimes the reinforcer might be a short break to play with a favorite toy while you catch your breath and set up the next activity.

Expect that he may be very resistant at first and throw toys or bite the toys, himself or you. This situation is new, and therefore alarming to Darius, and it may take him a while to realize that the reinforcer results from the work being done and that there is satisfaction in seeing the completely assembled toy. You may have to physically help a lot at first and he may be resistant, but if the activities are developmentally appropriate and the reinforcers are strong, he will probably soon be eager to work with you.

Goal #2: Darius will engage in joint play with an adult for 15-minute sessions and will imitate two modeled actions and two modeled meaningful vocal sounds or words per session.

For Goal #2 you will sometimes be playing on the floor, so to keep his attention you may need to start in a small space with the door closed and just a few toys available. Sit with your back against the door if he tends to flee, and for a while just watch and try to join what Darius is doing. If all he's doing is trying to escape, you may have to spend a session or two just sharing a snack or lining up his cars. You may need a number of five-minute sessions initially, but always try to end when he is calm and you can be relaxed as you open the door and say "All done."

When he is comfortable in the space, start modeling simple play actions and a word or sound to go with them. Language models are your demonstrations of what Darius could say at that moment. You are hoping he will imitate exactly what you just said, so your models should be at, and just slightly above, his current level of speech, not matched to his assumed level of understanding. Play models are similar. You are showing him something he can do with a toy and hoping he will imitate you, so it should not be complex. If he later does it spontaneously, without you doing or saying it first, that's even better progress.

A language model provides the word that matches the concept the child is experiencing, giving him a sample to imitate. It is important to match the timing of your words to what Darius is doing or watching you do. Use modeling in routines such as eating, bathing and dressing as well as during play. Even if he is not yet ready to say the word, hearing an adult say it as he experiences it helps him develop his understanding of speech.

Some play and language modeling examples for Darius

As he is lining up his cars, say "More" as he reaches for another one and "Car" as he picks it up and "Car" again as he puts it in the line.

Make a tower, saying "More" as you reach for the next block, "On" as you place it on the tower and "Uh-oh!" when the tower falls.

Model meaningful sounds as well as words. "Uh-oh" is one example. Others might be "Mmm" when he's eating something he really likes, "Ow!" when he scrapes his knee, "Whee!" as he whirls in a circle, "Uh!" when he's pulling on something. You could model "Uh!" as you pretend to struggle to pull apart large pop-beads or plastic eggs. Then drop the pieces in a bucket, saying "In" as you let go of each one. If Darius grabs and dumps the bucket, you say "Dump!" as he does so.

Hold a wrapping-paper tube at a slant, put one of his cars in the top end, saying "In" as you do so, and then say "Go!" and let the car go down the tube. If he seems to be ignoring you, do the same action a half dozen times then set it aside and try something else. Next time, or the time after that, he may join you or even initiate the action himself because it is now familiar.

Modeling language in daily routines

If Darius indicates nonverbally that he wants more of something, like food, a toss in the air or a squeeze, say "More!" or "Again!" and then immediately give him the item or do the action. As you push him on a swing, say "Push!" as an instruction to yourself just before you push him. After a few repetitions of this, pause to see if he will vocalize or say an approximation of "Push" to ask you to do it again.

When Darius wants something and you are sure you know what he wants, such as Cheerios™, but he is not trying to say it, take advantage of his attention to model it several times as you get it for him. For example, say "Cheerios...want Cheerios" (or just "Ohs" to make it easier for him to say) as you take the box from the shelf, again as you pour some in a bowl and as you pause before giving it to him. You are not refusing to give it to him unless he says it; you are just making sure he hears the name of the thing he wants several times. If he tries to say "Oh" or "Cheerio," repeat it back and quickly give him some.

Point to and name pictures in a word book, the ones that just have pictures of common objects with labels under them. Use the same few pages for several sessions if he ignores or avoids books. Many young children on the autism spectrum can't follow a story but will pay attention to a word book used for labeling pictures. Even if Darius ignores it for a while, he is likely to become more attentive if he hears you name the same few pictures a number of different times.

The most important thing to remember is that you are doing the actions and saying the sounds or words that Darius could do or say in that situation (not telling him what to do) and providing models that are only a little bit more advanced than his present speech.

Goal #3: Darius will request specific pieces of three different inset-style puzzles by pointing to each piece in a photograph of the completed puzzle. In a reversed activity, he will give an adult the specific pieces which the adult requests by naming and pointing to the piece in the photo.

Remember, Darius already has demonstrated the ability to make requests by giving an adult a picture of the thing he wants, so it may be fairly easy for him to learn to also make requests by pointing to one item in a more complex picture, as one would do when selecting from a picture menu in a restaurant or pointing out desired items in a toy catalogue. For this activity, I typically use puzzles in which each piece has a name, sits in its own hole and depicts a common object such as a farm animal, vehicle, number or shape. It provides another opportunity for modeling the single-word names of the pieces as he requests them and again as you hand them to him. Therefore, while working on this goal, you are also addressing his first two goals.

This activity works on pointing as an alternative means of choosing, not as a replacement for picture exchange. Since it is a clear, structured routine, Darius should easily do it with another child once he is familiar with it.

Select one or more inset-style puzzles (each piece has its own hole in the puzzle board), with four or more pieces. Print a good clear photo of each completed puzzle, which can be as big as the puzzle itself or as small as four by six inches, depending on his vision and dexterity. Darius needs to be able to see the individual pieces of the puzzle clearly in the photo and point to one piece without his finger overlapping onto another piece in the photo. A five-by-seven-inch photo of the completed puzzle might be a good starting size for Darius.

Have some small treats as reinforcers if you need to help him stay focused on the activity. If used, these should be given immediately after a desired response, whether his action is spontaneous or assisted by the prompter. Have one adult to do the activity with Darius and, ideally, another adult to silently prompt him. One adult can do both, but it may be difficult at first.

This activity can be done with Darius requesting puzzle pieces (expressive version) or the adult requesting the pieces (receptive version).

Procedure for the expressive version

Sit beside or across from Darius and present a puzzle that is familiar to him. You take the pieces and give Darius the empty puzzle board and the photo. Say/sign/gesture "What do you want?" indicating the photo as you speak.

Darius points to one of the puzzle pieces in the photo of the completed puzzle, or is assisted to do so, preferably by another, silent adult sitting behind him. You name and give him the piece he chose and let him—or help him if necessary—put it in the puzzle.

Continue until the puzzle is completed. Feel free to help Darius put the pieces in if necessary to avoid frustration or distraction from the choosing process. If you have puzzles that you have already been working with as part of Goal #1 or 2, this will probably go smoothly. If you haven't worked with puzzles, you may want to do that for a while first, or try some of these tips:

- Initially, you or the other adult may need to slide the photo away and the puzzle closer after the Darius makes a choice, or otherwise move materials around to make it easier.

- Starting with a four-piece puzzle or covering some of the puzzle parts in the photo may help if there are too many choices or Darius is requesting pieces he has already put in the puzzle.

- You may need to gently help him shape his hand into a one-finger point if he taps the photo with all his fingers extended.

- If he points to a piece in the photo that has already been put in the puzzle, say "(Name of piece) is all done," point to it in the puzzle, repeat "What do you want?" and have the prompter help him choose one that isn't done. However, I have often been impressed with how readily children learn to do this activity without asking for pieces they already have.

- Give as much help as is needed to move through the process smoothly rather than letting Darius make, and try to correct, errors. Then gradually reduce the help as the process is learned.

Some children can easily shift between doing this activity receptively and expressively, but others may be quite confused if you do this. I would focus on having Darius be the requester (expressive version) until that is very familiar and then shift roles.

In the receptive version, which provides valuable practice in understanding vocabulary and following instructions, Darius has the loose pieces and the adult, who has the puzzle board and the photo, points to a specific puzzle piece in the photo and says, with hand extended, palm up, "I want the cow/circle/five," naming the requested piece. Darius finds and gives the correct piece, with the silent prompter helping as needed. With practice, he will probably learn to respond when you only say the name of the piece you want, without pointing to the photo.

Arnie could also learn to do this activity, though he would struggle with the receptive version if you stopped using the photo. Both the expressive and receptive versions would help increase his use of picture communication. It would be more challenging, but potentially possible for Rebecca too. It would help develop her ability to match pictures to identical objects, a skill she needs to progress from three-dimensional to two-dimensional communication systems. I learned this activity from a little nonverbal girl named Monica. She spontaneously began to point to specific puzzle pieces in a four-by-six-inch photo when I was only expecting her to point to the whole photo to request more pieces.

Accomplishing these three goals will help Darius interact productively with teachers while building his problem-solving skills with toys, introducing concepts such as recurrence (more), location (in, on) and action (go, push). He will also be increasing his ability to express desires with specific pointing and spoken words, comment on his activities and express basic feelings vocally (Ow, Mmm, Uh-oh, Whee!).

As we help Arnie and Darius improve their understanding and use of spoken language, we are also strengthening their shared attention, cognition and non-oral communication.

Chapter 4

Pre-Symbolic Communication and Emerging Speech: Expanded

When speech is a "not yet" skill for a prolonged time, communication is still vitally important. For children like Rebecca, Arnie and Darius, autism is accompanied by severe limitations in the understanding and use of spoken language and conventional gestures or manual signs. They need to develop basic functional communication. Parents worry about how people will know their non-speaking children's needs and wishes when the parents are not there to interpret. The goals highlighted in the last two chapters were chosen to address some of these early communication issues.

Expressive communication

Requesting and choosing, whether with speech or an alternative form of communication such as signing or picture exchange, are early communication functions which are very motivating to the child, require interaction with others and usually help begin to decrease problem behaviors. It is likely that the child already has a sense of "wanting," which makes it easier to develop a means of expressing that concept in a way that is more conventional and desirable than screaming. Other, more social, communicative functions typically seen in the gestures of pre-verbal toddlers, such as waving a greeting or pointing out things they notice or need help with, are less likely to be in the spontaneous repertoire of pre-symbolic children on the autism spectrum. This means the children would need to learn the underlying concept or intent of the message as well as the words to express the meanings. And some of the things parents especially want their children to communicate, such as feelings, yes/no answers or the need to use the toilet, are often beyond the comprehension level of this group.

Rebecca, Arnie and Darius are all using some form of requesting by exchanging a symbol for a desired item. For Rebecca, this occurs mainly as a scheduled opportunity, although her board is also available to her throughout the day. Arnie needs to be prompted to make a choice, except for his ketchup. Darius is the most independent of the three because he will go to his board, select a symbol and then seek a parent so he can deliver it. All of their systems can be used at school and at home, and can be expanded to include many more options. The boys using picture symbols could probably transition easily to a basic speech-generating device (SGD). Their present levels of language do not suggest readiness for creating sentences with strips of pictures or an SGD, but further progress should be expected.

People sometimes wonder if teaching alternative means of communication will make it less likely that the child will learn to talk, but research consistently shows that this is not the case (Millar, Light and Schlosser 2006). Anecdotally, consider Darius, whose first few spoken words are the names of things on his choice board.

Receptive communication

Understanding simple instructions and recognizing the names of common objects can increase safety, help the child understand his environment, and promote recognition of communication as a two-way street. Arnie's goals of learning to come, give and wait relate to easing safety concerns, but vigilant supervision is still a must. Learning the names of common functional objects and action verbs like "put," "take" and "open" will support his knowledge of the world, his life skills learning and his educational progress.

Darius has goals for learning to take instruction, focus his attention, play in meaningful and productive ways, and develop a repertoire of things he can do by himself instead of aimless wandering and climbing. Through modeling, which matches the names of toys and actions to his immediate experiences, he is increasing his understanding of language, and for the words he imitates orally, increasing his expressive vocabulary.

Some other useful skills to teach

Here are a few examples of some additional possible goals for these three children and others at a similar developmental level:

- Following an adult's finger point as an instruction to "Put it here" with puzzles or objects, as a direction to sit in a chair or an indication to look at something.

- Following a familiar multi-step routine with picture schedule support. Examples might be gathering articles of clothing before dressing or finding a bowl, spoon and box of cereal for breakfast. For a short routine sequence like hand washing or tooth brushing, I typically do not recommend a series of steps on a picture schedule because I believe that interrupting the flow of action to refer to the schedule interferes with the development of procedural memory, the unconscious, long-term memory of how to do familiar tasks. Nonverbal prompting and elimination of stops and starts makes it easier for the child to learn the flow of a routine process.

- Understanding that pictures can support instructions so the child knows that if you show him a picture of his coat and say "Get your coat," that is an instruction, but when he gives you a picture, he is requesting an object or action from you. When the connection between pictures and the objects they represent is solid, nonverbal children are better able to participate in joint play, book sharing and activities like retrieving their clothing on request or gathering specific items from a picture list.

* Using pointing as well as picture exchange to indicate wants, with picture boards or speech-generating devices. This might include pointing to specific pieces of a puzzle, food items on a picture menu or a choice of movies. The process for teaching this with puzzles is described in Chapter 3 in the section on Darius's Goal #3.

* Responding to a high five as a greeting or signing "please" to mean "I want." Signs and gestures that make contact with the body are often easier to learn than those that occur in the air, such as waving or signing "want."

* Learning to imitate actions with objects (like activating a noise-making toy or piling blocks) and actions without objects (like clapping or waving). This can progress to imitation of meaningful sounds (like "Mmm, Uh-oh, Whee!") and simple words. Aim for words that are easier to say and will be useful in the child's life, but also consider strong interests. One little boy's first 30 "words" included 22 letters of the alphabet because he was strongly attracted to print. While not highly functional for earliest communication, many letter names are good for articulation practice. Expect to practice verbal imitation repeatedly with strong reinforcers, and alternate easier imitations with more difficult ones to maintain the child's motivation.

* Doing with a classmate some of the table activities he has learned to do with an adult. This will involve more pre-teaching/coaching of the classmate than of the child on the autism spectrum. If the peer just takes the adult's role and does the activity in the same way the child learned it, the autistic child will usually respond as he has practiced.

- Completing progressively more complicated problem-solving tasks involving puzzles, matching, sorting and simple assembly. Often these may overlap nicely with goals of occupational therapy or early education.

- Following a basic sequence of *independent work*. This will be described more fully in Chapter 6 but is often a productive activity for pre-symbolic students as well.

Key points about teaching methods

Create a one-to-one teaching structure

As described in Chapter 3 for Darius's first goal, establish a place and a system for direct instruction, starting with simple, toy-based learning that you can physically help him to do and then immediately reinforce. Between activities, you may need to slide the new work in front of him as you remove the one that he just completed. Otherwise, he may disappear while you are reaching for a puzzle.

Most autistic children will come willingly to a learning session and wait between activities, when they realize that the expectations are doable, satisfying and rewarded. Some even cry when a session ends. Because play sessions will be less structured and may not involve treats, it may be important to play in a confined space so the child does not just leave.

In the previous two chapters, I have frequently recommended using few words and prompting nonverbally. If this seems stern or unfriendly to you, please be assured that it is not meant to be. If you see yourself as helping rather than coercing, and stay calm and unhurried, you can convey reassurance and encouragement without words. In fact, you can often be more supportive and communicative with fewer words.

Use visual schedules

Everyone who works with students on the autism spectrum is probably familiar with the use of visual schedules. Nearly all programs use them.

Usually, they are created because they provide the predictability, routine and security that autism craves, resulting in fewer behavioral problems. Many tasks are more readily completed because they are on the schedule, and referring to a schedule also often helps the student transition more smoothly to the next activity.

For children in the pre-symbolic range of development, the items on the schedule can be represented by objects, photos or pictures/symbols, preferably with the words adults should call them written underneath the symbols.

Use a simple script with the schedule:

"Check the schedule." "Bathroom is done/finished" (you or the child pull off the symbol and put it in a box).

"Time for snack" (tapping the symbol as you say this).

If trying to schedule major events of the day seems daunting, try just using the schedule for individual teaching sessions at first. Even a simple "work-work-choice" routine can be helpful. A lesson plan can be represented by something as simple as two square buttons to represent learning tasks and a round button for choice. Initially, you will be saying "work one...work one is done...work two..." and so on as you remove buttons and drop them into a box, with the child paying no apparent attention and possibly trying to flee. But the repetition will be predictable and comforting, and he will probably soon be helping you, or at least waiting calmly, while you set up the next activity.

Schedules are not outgrown; they grow up with the child. Later, they can be valuable for teaching flexibility and independence.

Just start

If shifting between learning activities is difficult, move past the transition as smoothly as possible. Just start doing a familiar, less demanding activity yourself, and the autistic child will often join you. Even if you need to help him more than usual at the beginning of the activity, the "Just start" procedure creates a valuable bridge to cooperation. I have found it to be much more effective than waiting and trying to establish that the child is ready to participate. If he is likely to dash away when arriving at the teaching session, have the materials, and the reinforcer, ready before he arrives, and begin with something you can physically assist him to do, such as a puzzle or shape sorter. To shorten the transition between activities, you may need to slide the new work in front of him as you remove the completed task.

Reinforce the behaviors you want to see again

If you ask Arnie to give you the spoon, and he does so, reinforce that action quickly with "Spoon!" and a treat. But if he gives you the spoon and then sweeps the other items off the table before you have responded, don't give the reward or you will be reinforcing the behavior of sweeping items off the table. Just do the task again and reinforce quickly, even if you helped. A reinforcer increases the chances that the immediately preceding action of the child will occur again, so be sure that the child will associate the reward with the action you want him to repeat.

Keep calm and carry on

If the child is agitated, upset or otherwise rambunctious, stay quiet and predictable, and try to get the task back on track without raising your voice or giving reassurances, warnings and treat reminders, or even appearing to be bothered. Take a few turns yourself, saying what you would say if he did it ("Circle...it's in!") and even popping a treat in your own mouth. Help him do a simple task with hand-over-hand assistance and reward as if he did it himself, then gradually reduce your help over the next few turns.

If all else fails, try to get one good response, even if for a simpler task ("Clap your hands"), reward that response, say "All done!" and let him go. If he has already bolted and is gone, try again later, starting with some expectations you know he can meet easily or activities you know he enjoys. I do not believe it is worth fighting to keep the child working because the struggle can quickly become a habit and autistic children will often behave in ways that maintain a predictable pattern even if it is negative for everyone. That is, he may resist again next time just because he did this time. In the long run, short positive sessions will carry more value than long embattled ones, even if you win the battle. Try to end a teaching session when the child is working well with you. *Aim for cooperation rather than compliance.*

Use errorless learning when possible

This is another way of saying "Teach, don't test." Most of the teaching activities I recommend involve helping the child respond correctly rather than allowing for and correcting mistakes. Visual supports and physical prompts are very helpful here.

A simple example is Arnie's task to give an object from a group of four on the table. If you ask him "Give me the shoe" four times and three of those times he gives you a different object, he has practiced being wrong three out of four times and was probably only correct the other time by chance. So he has heard you say "shoe" while he is looking at a spoon or cup or whatever incorrect item he gave you. Even if you stop and correct him each time, he is more likely to be confused than if he just gets it right the first time he hears it.

But if you show him another shoe, or picture of a shoe, to match with the one you request, he is much more likely to be correct. If he is not, you will help him reach for the right one. By responding correctly, even with all that help, he has seen a shoe while hearing the word "shoe" at least three times, increasing the chances that he will learn the word and become able to respond without the visual cue. And if he doesn't learn the spoken word, he will be developing an understanding that a picture cue can be used to help him interpret a message. This too is a very valuable communication skill.

Don't assume comprehension

It is true that children developing language typically understand more language than they can use expressively, but developmentally young children on the autism spectrum often don't give us the nonverbal clues that indicate they understand us, such as retrieving items we ask for or smiling and clapping in response to hearing "Pizza for supper!" If team members judge comprehension based on clear, observable behaviors rather than on assumptions without evidence, they will be less likely to blame the child for non-compliance when the actual problem is non-comprehension. For the child's sake, and for realistic planning, it is better if you are a bit skeptical and assume he might not have understood.

If the child in question does demonstrate strong comprehension skills but is unable to produce much recognizable speech, the possibility of dyspraxia should be considered. It is, of course, also possible to have a motor speech disability such as dyspraxia or dysarthria and autism and poor comprehension, just as it is possible to have autism with blindness, deafness, cerebral palsy or a mental illness, but those complications are mainly beyond the scope of this book.

Model the language the child could be saying

Language modeling is a method of pairing the concepts a child is experiencing with the words that express them. It involves providing a sample to the child of the words that go with what he's doing. Essentially, the parent talks for the child, commenting on objects and events from the child's point of view.

It is not questions, instructions, explanations, praise or requests to "Say..." All these techniques have their uses, but they are not models. Models are examples of what the child could say at that moment. You are hoping he will imitate exactly what you just said, and even if he doesn't, you will be encouraging comprehension by matching spoken words to his immediate experiences.

Language modeling provides a child with the symbols (words and/or signs) which represent the concepts he is discovering. Young children learn a great deal from their own activities, especially their play, and their earliest language reflects what they know about the world. For example, they learn that people and objects can disappear ("all gone") and recur ("more"), that they have names ("Mommy," "book"), can move and be moved ("go," "push"), have meaningful characteristics ("hot," "broken"), can have and change locations ("up," "in"), can be rejected ("no!") or possessed ("Mommy's," "mine!") and so on.

Examples of ways to combine language modeling and play development can be found in Chapter 3 in the description of Darius's second goal.

A language model provides the word that matches the concept the child is experiencing, giving him a sample to imitate. Even if he is not yet ready to say the word, hearing an adult say it as he experiences it helps him develop his understanding of speech and concepts.

Some points to remember about language modeling

+ You need to be doing something to talk about, and children learn from their play, so developing shared attention to activities and simple play skills is an important part of early language modeling.

+ Reduce the length and complexity of what you say to a level at or just a bit above what the child uses, not at or above what he understands. If he's not talking at all, single words and meaningful non-words ("Mmm, Ahhh! Whee!") are best.

+ Be brief but use acceptable grammar. It's better for you to say "Daddy's shoe" even if you know the child will reduce the possessive form to "Daddy shoe" or just "Daddy" and a pat on the shoe.

+ Be repetitive. Don't worry about sounding boring or foolish because you say "in" 25 times while your child drops blocks in a can one at a time.

- Try to speak as the child acts. For example, say "up" as he goes up a step, "in" as he fits the piece into the puzzle or "book" as he picks one up. Talk more about what he is doing than what you are doing.

- Avoid encouraging funny sounds like "raspberries" or giggly squeals or vocalizations that the child repeats frequently but without apparent meaning. These may be cute now but very hard to un-teach later.

- Recognize that you are also modeling language during the structured teaching sessions described in this book, such as when you say "shoe" three times during a sorting task, and that the child may pay closer attention in a structured session. But it is important to model language in more natural play and daily living situations too.

For some children with delayed speech development, language modeling and their own developmental maturation will be sufficient to establish communicative speech in words and phrases, but for children on the autism spectrum it will probably be one of many therapy techniques.

Prompt nonverbally

In the previous chapters, I frequently mentioned having a silent partner help prompt a child to avoid the confusion of two people talking. When a person does not understand language well, hearing more of it is not often helpful, especially if two adults are talking at once. Even if you are working alone with your child, fewer words, supported by a gentle nudge or other physical prompt, will often be more effective than multiple repetitions or rewording of messages. Some people talk more and faster when attempting to calm a child who is upset, confused or uncooperative. Try not to be one of those people.

Nonverbal prompting is also important in developing independence in activities such as hand washing, exchanging a request symbol or eating with a spoon because it is more easily faded than verbal prompts. You can gradually decrease nonverbal prompts from full assistance to partial help, to just a nudge on an elbow as the child becomes more independent.

Behavior

Recognize the difficulties the child brings to the situation as a result of a neurologically based disorder. Although some behavioral upsets are the result of unmet desires, many stem from the anxiety inherent in having autism in a neurotypical world. Among the common characteristics of these children, which often lead to behavioral conflicts, are the following:

- ✦ Significant, atypical difficulties with understanding and using language, especially in group situations. This is exacerbated if educational expectations are beyond the child's current ability.

- ✦ Often, an overly reactive sensory system that makes ordinary noise, smell or touch irritating or intolerable.

- ✦ Problems shifting attention or "transitioning" from one activity to another.

- ✦ Limited ability to recognize another person's perspective or opinion or to empathize with another's feelings.

- ✦ A need for predictability and routine, and a tendency to respond based on association and memory. These characteristics lead the child to repeat familiar behaviors even when they produce consistently negative results.

- ✦ Poor recognition of public vs. private behavior and limited embarrassment or concern about other people's impressions of them. Or, if they are concerned, they may have little ability to repair the interaction.

◆ Emotional responses that are apt to be extreme and are often based on immediate events, leading to rapid changes from smiling to screaming. Emotional recovery may be immediate once the problem is removed, but for some children irritability and secondary upsets can continue for hours.

◆ Considerable difficulty organizing themselves to do something productive in undirected play activities, in stimulating public situations or when waiting.

◆ Problems with sleep, diet, sensory responses, anxiety and life skills can improve with growth in communication, but often continue to be difficult for even the most linguistically advanced people on the autism spectrum.

Remember, these struggles are not the result of poor parenting or teaching, nor are they deliberate, willful or manipulative behaviors. They are simply common characteristics of children on the autism spectrum and they are nobody's fault. These behavioral characteristics are also true of the children in the two other groups in this book, although they may be manifested differently.

It is important when working with pre-symbolic children to stay calm but alert, minimize confusing language, have strong reinforcers, use visual schedules and errorless learning, and teach the early developing behaviors of choosing, requesting, direction following and play skills.

Tracking progress

Opinions differ on how to track progress in educational programs and on how much information is enough. But we can probably agree that it is important to know if what we are doing is working.

Schools and programs may have established systems they want their whole team to follow but, as with the writing of goals, they don't all do it the same way. And, like the specifics of goal writing, the particulars of data collection are not a major focus of this book.

In my experience, tracking progress in communication requires some flexibility depending on the type of goal being assessed. Spontaneous communications in natural settings can't be measured the same way as responses in structured teaching sessions.

For example, to assess Rebecca's progress on approaching someone to nonverbally request a share of something (Goal #2), you might record whether she needed assistance to do the various parts of the communication. List the components on a form:

- approached the person

- extended her hand

- turned her hand palm up.

Mark each with an "S" if she did it spontaneously and a "P" (for prompt) if you had to physically help her. Later, you could add signing "please" as a fourth component.

When Arnie is practicing "Give me the..." (Goal #3), list the items you could ask for and record a "+" or "-" to indicate whether he responded correctly. Do ten of these requests and it is easy to determine a percentage correct. You will also have data on which words are becoming more familiar to him.

Record the date and length of time for the play session (Goal #2) with Darius and note any actions or words he imitates. Add a check mark for every extra time he imitates the same word or action during a session. If he uses a previously modeled play action or word without you doing it first, circle it to indicate that it was spontaneous. This would be a good job for an observer or to transcribe from a video, so you can focus fully on Darius.

These are over-simplifications, of course. Among other factors, you might need to know if you helped a little or a lot, whether any unpleasant behaviors were involved or which toys were being used.

You also need to be able to explain what the results indicate. For example, "Rebecca can now reliably (80% of opportunities) approach an adult holding a snack or toy Rebecca likes and reach out, but not grab the item. She still frequently needs a light touch on her hand as a prompt to turn her hand so her palm is facing up."

But the key points are: Know what you are measuring, know where you started, use a system that interferes minimally with your teaching, and know what progress is occurring.

Generalization

Few goals are really functional if they can only be demonstrated in a structured practice situation. To be independent in these early skills, a child should make requests without adult prompting, use toys outside of teaching sessions, respond to known directions and vocabulary in natural settings, and say things spontaneously, not just when told to say them. Getting there will require lots of practice in real situations with teachers, parents and peers.

These children will also need accommodations such as fidget toys, sensory aids, abbreviated community outings and perhaps cards explaining autism for parents to give to alarmed strangers.

Parents, teachers and children dealing with autism usually are doing the best they can and deserve tolerance, acceptance and encouragement from others they encounter.

What if they are already adults?

Sometimes, autistic people reach adulthood without developing a useful means of communication. The first priority then is establishing a safe, comfortable living environment that is as stable as possible and provides a good quality of life. But learning does not need to stop with the end of school. Many of the basic skills of object and picture communication, for making requests, waiting and following instructions are still worth pursuing, as are skills in using objects appropriately, with an emphasis on self-help, domestic and recreational activities in place of toys.

The bottom line

For a pre-symbolic child or adult on the autism spectrum, learning will be a long, effortful process and most of it will be directed by others. Given this dependence on time and hard work, it is very important to carefully choose and work on goals that the person has the developmental ability to accomplish, that are useful now and in the future, and that will improve his safety, happiness, independence and productivity.

PART II

ATYPICAL LANGUAGE

Chapter 5

Echolalia

Lucas

As a child's language emerges, and he begins to say a lot of single words and short phrases, we expect to hear progressively more varied vocabulary, longer and more complex sentences, and considerably more conversation. And we expect this advancing language to be used for functional communication and social interaction and as a gateway to lots of new learning.

Some children on the autism spectrum do make rapid progress after learning to talk but most continue to need help. There are many ways to work on expanding communication skills at home, in school or through speech and language therapy in groups or individual sessions. At this point, many autistic children respond well to teaching methods similar to those provided to children with language delays and disorders that are not complicated by autism. However, the autistic child will benefit from therapy sessions with a predictable routine and a visual schedule and will probably require more help with some aspects of communication, such as understanding non-literal language like idioms and sarcasm, reading (especially fiction) with comprehension, and conversing and interacting socially. Also, autism does not insulate a child from other possible communication difficulties such as hearing loss, stuttering, voice disorders or problems articulating speech clearly.

However, many children on the autism spectrum, even without any additional speech and language problems, develop language on a more divergent path known as echolalia.

Echolalia is a fascinating, challenging and sometimes frustrating language disorder that often accompanies autism spectrum disorders. I have known quite a few congenitally blind or visually impaired children with echolalia. They have always shown additional characteristics of autism and are increasingly being given diagnoses on the autism spectrum. The echolalia of some of the visually impaired children has been especially striking because they were talking excessively and speaking very clearly.

Echolalic language is heavily based on immediate or delayed repetition of phrases and sentences other people have just said or that the child has previously heard someone say in similar situations.

Immediate echoes

Mother: Do you want cereal or pancakes?

Daughter: Cereal or pancakes?

Neighbor: Good morning, Samantha.

Child: Good morning, Samantha.

Delayed echoes

Mother to son: Get in the car. I need to pick up your sister.

Father: (the next morning as the family is going out for breakfast) Get in the car.

Son: I need to pick up your sister.

Child: (hearing cupboard doors opening, or perhaps just wanting a snack) Do you want a cookie?

Characteristics of echolalic communication include difficulty with language comprehension, confusion of pronouns, overuse of a questioning intonation and very compromised ability to use speech to easily meet conversational needs. Children who echo are attempting to use speech for functional communicative purposes, such as requesting, directing, protesting, commenting, or even just taking a conversational turn, but it is often up to the listener to interpret the child's apparent meaning.

Echolalia typically goes with excellent auditory memory, limited and repetitive play skills, and impaired social interaction. Behavioral challenges often include automatic and extreme resistance to changes, transitions and new experiences, as well as perseverative self-stimulating actions, poor safety awareness and atypical eating and sleeping patterns. In other words, echolalia goes with autism.

The therapeutic process, as I see it, involves working on functional expressive communication, cognitive development, language comprehension, play skills and social interaction. Where to start depends on the child's present level, but it is important not to assume that strong memory, and sometimes oral reading skills, are indicative of the child's actual cognitive and language development. It may appear that the child's expressive use of language is more advanced than his comprehension, but true novel expressive language requires a more solid base of understanding language than is typical with echolalia. The goal of intervention is not to eliminate echolalia by teaching the child to repress it, but to replace it with conventional language so he no longer needs it.

Here are some communication issues that usually need to be addressed:

• Reversal of personal pronouns (using you/your/yours for I/me/my/mine).

• Excessive use of questions "Do you want...?" in place of requests like "I want..." and as comments ("It's a big one?") and an intonation pattern in which most of the child's speech sounds like questions.

+ Little ability to answer or ask true questions.

+ An automatic "No!" response when asked to do something or transition to another activity or when offered something new. Although many don't say "yes," some children who echo will only answer "yes" and are very resistant to saying "no."

+ Perseverating on saying certain phrases over and over.

+ Reciting (sometimes repeatedly) lines from movies or books that are at best tangentially related to the present situation and have no obvious communicative intent.

+ Echoing praise, greetings and protests exactly as heard.

Children who have been echolalic but have progressed to more conventional speech and language have some typical characteristics which are also common among verbal autistic children who have not been echolalic. These include:

+ strong memory, rote learning and associative skills, but difficulty with verbal reasoning or flexible thought

+ concrete literal interpretation of language

+ oral reading that is significantly more advanced than reading comprehension

+ difficulty using memorized information in new ways and generalizing learned skills to new situations

+ excessive questioning, sometimes just to get a known, predictable answer

+ poor understanding of the meaning carried in gestures, eye gaze and intonation patterns

- difficulty following group discussions, repairing communication breakdowns, shifting topics and recognizing and responding to the interests and ideas of others

- extreme interest in, and desire to talk about, narrow topics, usually those that can be memorized and classified such as road maps, sport statistics and movies, but sometimes those that are alarming and beyond an individual's control like violent weather or death

- possibly, strong "savant" skills and talents in areas like music, art or mathematical calculation that are much more advanced than the child's other abilities.

In the rest of this chapter and in Chapter 6 some of these concerns will be described and discussed through the stories of three children, Lucas and Seth, who have significant echolalia, and Terek, who has been developing language without echolalia.

Lucas

Lucas is three and a half years old. He talks in phrases and sentences but does not truly converse. He most frequently speaks to make requests and does so by saying the words used by people offering things to him. For example, if he wants to use the boat in his preschool, he says "(Do) you wanta use the boat?" If he's thirsty, he says "Do you want a drink?" and he says "Help you?" to mean "I need help." When parting from his parents at the preschool door, he echoes "Have a good day at school" as they are leaving.

When people greet him by name, he either repeats "Hi Lucas" or says nothing at all. If someone tells him "No" or "Don't..." Lucas is likely to say "Don't touch the microwave!" in an alarmed tone of voice, because he associates any prohibition with the one he hears most often at home. Much of his speech has a questioning intonation because he is remembering and reusing the language forms adults most often use to address him, and adults ask children lots of questions. Lucas responds to most offers or suggestions of activities such as "Can you...?" or "Do you want to...?" with a very quick, automatic and determined "No?" Like much of his speech, this "no" sounds like a question but it is often an emphatic refusal, sometimes paired with pulling away. He never says the word "yes," nor does he use other affirmation words like "sure" and "okay." If asked a question such as "Did you have fun at school?" he may flap his hands, hop in place and say "Fun at school? You have fun at school?"

Like many children who echo language, Lucas tends to say things that he has heard in a similar situation but which do not quite match his actions or his role in the conversation, such as the following:

- Saying "Are you finished?" or "Are you all done?" when he means he wants to end an activity. At his pediatrician's office he attempts to escape by saying repeatedly "Say bye Doctor! Say bye Doctor!" because his mother usually prompts him to "Say goodbye to the doctor" as they are leaving.

- Repeating some of the more unusual or dramatic things he has heard previously, at random times and without an observable connection, such as "Silly goose!" and "That's enough!" Since his big sister said "Oooh, gas!" once after Lucas expelled some, he frequently giggles and says "Oooh, gas!" at random, or sometimes embarrassing, times.

- Saying "Here we go!" repeatedly as he continues to sit at the top of the slide while a crowd of waiting children gathers on the steps behind him.

Lucas knows the words to several children's songs, but rarely sings in unison. He will sing alone (not necessarily when requested) or fill in words if a partner stops singing, but he tends to just listen when a group of others are singing.

He looks for patterns in language and seems to be actively trying to associate words with their meanings. Sometimes his questions seem appropriate, such as when he asked "Where's the big mirror?" as he went to it, but he did not appear to be expecting an answer, clearly knew where the mirror was, and was actually echoing a question his teacher had asked the day before.

Lucas has limited play skills and a tendency toward repetitive manipulation of objects, like his long spells of opening and closing the toy barn doors, turning the lights on and off a dozen times in a row at home, and filling every hole in a pegboard. He does have a great interest in his magnetic letters of the alphabet and anything in print, and at age three and a half he has spontaneously learned to read without instruction. He reads road signs, his father's co-workers' name tags, grocery flyers and car brands. He does not appear to understand simple stories, whether he reads them himself or someone reads to him. This unusual reading ability is known as hyperlexia and occurs fairly often with autism.

He prefers to interact with adults rather than children, probably because adults are more predictable and accommodating, and therefore "safer" and less confusing.

In summary, Lucas's emerging language is significantly echolalic, with the accompanying characteristics of strong auditory memory, delayed language comprehension, very limited play skills, poor peer interaction and avoidance of unfamiliar activities. He attempts to take his conversational turn, make requests, affirm, protest or refuse verbally, comment on activities or conversation and respond to questions, but he does these things by reusing whole chunks of language he has heard, memorized and associated with the present moment. He lacks true comprehension of the questions, conversation or explanations that would be understood by his age-mates.

We will consider four goals for Lucas that focus on beginning to use personal pronouns, increasing meaningful play and language that matches it, responding to greetings without echoing and interacting with other children.

Goal #1: Lucas will spontaneously make requests for objects in the form "I want..." and direct actions by saying "Please..." in three practice settings and four or more times per day in naturally occurring situations.

This goal addresses two language functions, requesting tangible items such as food or a toy and requesting action from another person such as help or a push in a swing. Lucas would probably request a cookie by saying "Do you want a cookie?" or perhaps even "Do you want a cookie? Say please!" He clearly expects to eat that cookie himself even though he sounds as if he is offering it to you.

For clarity, I refer to requesting an action as "directing." When looking for assistance while putting on boots, his echoed directive might be "Need help?" or "Do you need some help?" or "Can you do it all by yourself?" All of these would be memorized chunks, delayed echoes of things adults have said to him in similar situations.

In these examples, he is motivated to communicate and the language is functional to him, but it requires interpretation by the listener. Attempting to explain to Lucas that I say "I" when I mean myself and you say "I" when you mean yourself will simply get us both into deep conversational weeds.

If we can shift the two early developing and frequently used communicative functions of requesting and directing to more conventional forms, Lucas, and other children who echo, will be more readily understood, will begin to see how conversational roles shift with different speakers, and will practice language forms that can be a learning platform for creating other novel sentences. We will also make a dent in his excessively questioning intonation. Let's begin with "I want."

Requesting

Start by expecting just a single-word request, the name of the desired item. Show Lucas something you know he likes, such as a piece of apple, and say "Apple!" but hold on to it if he tries to grab it. You say "Apple!" again once or twice with pauses between, and give it to him whether he echoes it or not. Since he echoes readily, he will probably start imitating "Apple" after a few rounds of this as he discovers that he gets it more quickly that way. Any time he echoes "Apple" or says it spontaneously, you quickly give him the apple piece as you say "Apple!" enthusiastically. Don't praise him or say that he can have the apple, as this is likely to add confusion and he may start echoing those words. You don't want Lucas to be saying "Good job!" or "Here's your apple" as he takes the apple. Likewise, this is not a good time to tell him to "Say apple" or he is apt to use "Sayapple" as a request instead of just "Apple." And, of course, don't ask him if he wants some apple as that is the echo we are trying to replace with a conventional request.

When Lucas is reliably imitating you, put longer pauses between your offers so he has an opportunity to ask without you saying it first. If he says "Apple" before you do, be sure to give it to him because this spontaneous request is more advanced than his imitation of you. Practice this with a variety of things he wants and that you can provide in small pieces or tiny sips. It could be toys like Lego™ or little cars if you know he will want more and keep asking for them. Pegs for his pegboard or his magnetic letters would work well. For most of these he can say the same word every time (Lego, car, peg) but with the letters have him imitate or spontaneously name the specific letter. Just avoid giving him something you let him use briefly and then have to take back so he will ask again. This may aggravate him. Offer things he can either consume or keep throughout the activity.

When he is spontaneously naming "Apple" or other items to get you to let go of them, you start saying "Want apple." If he just says "Apple," you repeat "Want apple" one or two times and then give it to him, but he will probably start saying "Want apple" fairly soon. We know that remembering a two-word combination is no challenge for Lucas and he echoes very readily. A less verbal child will take longer to go through this process.

The next step is to include "I" + "want" + "apple" and to help Lucas begin to see that "I" means the person who is speaking. Take his hand, gently bend all his fingers to point toward his chest and tap his fingers on his chest as you model "*I* want apple." Be sure to tap *only* as you say "I," not with each word in the sentence. The hand cue will be an important part of helping him learn that "I" means Lucas, so we want to associate it only with the word "I." Practice with the pegs, letters and other items at this level too, and if he omits the "I," try to cue him by just tapping his hand on his chest. If he doesn't immediately respond to the hand cue, you can whisper "I," but he may just finish with "want apple."

Another motivating activity for practicing "I want..." and hearing that everyone uses it to refer to themselves is to have a shared snack. Find another adult or cooperative child to help you and gather three different snack items that can be given out in small pieces. For Lucas, apple would be one because he has already practiced asking for it, and the others might be grapes and small crackers. One helper says "I want a grape," the other helper says "Grape" and passes a grape or the dish of grapes. They each model this a few times, giving each other the requested snack food. Lucas may initially echo exactly what another person just requested but is very likely to spontaneously ask for his own preference soon. If not, you can prompt him as you did in the earlier practice, including the hand cue for "I," but this probably won't be necessary. Feel free to use more varied and complete requests like "some apple," "two grapes" or "more crackers," which were omitted earlier just to emphasize the key words.

But do keep the "I want..." format because we are building a foundation of "I" for self-reference with other verbs like "see," "found" and "am running." He could have easily learned to say "May I please have...?" instead of "I want," but it is a more advanced form of syntax and would be difficult to generalize to other uses.

In this context, I would save "please" and "thank you" for later as they are purely social words and can be confusing. Although adults naturally want to encourage politeness and autistic children clearly need help with social skills, the main goal here is understanding that "I" means self. "Please" can be more safely added to requests after the basic format is established. We will use "Please" as a starter word and a potential prompt in the next section on directing others.

"Thank you" is especially complicated. It must be said by the recipient, not the donor, after the request has been granted. "Thank you" is connected to no tangible referent and is usually followed by an equally unconnected social phrase, "You're welcome." I have often heard children saying "Thank you" as they hand something to someone else.

Because he has practiced it in a variety of natural situations, Lucas should start to use this "I want..." form of requesting in other situations fairly readily, but it does not mean that he truly understands that he should call himself "I." At this point it is a memorized chunk that works pretty well to get him what he wants. But he has practiced it a lot, associated the hand cue with the need to say "I" and heard other people saying the same words to obtain things they want, so it is a good start. We'll address using "I" more generally for self-reference in Goal #2.

Directing

Now let's consider directing, or asking another person to do something for him rather than to give him something.

Young children often need action from someone else to fix, open, zip, tie or push things or to just "help." Children on the autism spectrum often don't even realize that asking for help is an option and don't approach others for assistance. Lucas has learned that adults can help him but he echoes their words to signal his need and says things such as "Do you need help?" "Can you do it all by yourself?" and "Let me help you." He does not reliably approach an adult to say these things but may just fuss and say the words without directing them to a listener.

Since he doesn't directly request action from you, you'll need to physically prompt him. You, or a silent third person, seeing that he needs assistance, could help him hold out the ends of his jacket or a box he can't open and then you say "Please zip" or "Please open it" *as if directing yourself.* Don't say it with a questioning intonation like "Please open it?" or that's probably the way he'll say it too. You are modeling a polite imperative and Lucas will echo your intonation as well as your words.

If you know a particular directive is familiar to him, but he can't remember what to say right now, you can say "Please..." as a prompt and he may finish with "help," "zip it" or "open it." Again, be sure your "please" prompt does not have the rising intonation of a question. And be careful to avoid frequently responding "Okay" or "Mom will do it" after he directs you. Either do what he has asked without comment or give a variety of different responses, so he won't think he's supposed to repeat the whole thing, as in "Please zip it okay."

Goal #2: During guided play and daily-life activities, Lucas will reliably demonstrate the following functional communication behaviors with basic conventional, non-echolalic language:

+ commenting on his play and activities

+ using "I" as a subject pronoun with five different verbs

+ prohibiting others' actions

+ rejecting objects

+ making choices.

All of these can be worked on through language modeling, as described for Darius in Chapter 3, explained in more detail in Chapter 4, and presented here with variations for echolalia. It is still important to speak from the child's point of view and use language that is only slightly more advanced than the child uses, but there are some important variations for children who echo language.

Commenting

When playing with Lucas or helping him with dressing, eating, bathing and other one-to-one activities, avoid asking questions or giving verbal instructions that will sound strange if echoed. Instead, comment on the activity using words that would also be appropriate coming from Lucas and give physical assistance if necessary. For example, when helping him put nesting cups together, you could say something like:

"Cup goes in...another cup...uh-oh, too small...let's try this cup... there, it fits!"

During bathing you might say:

"Here's the washcloth...need some soap...gotta wash arms...washing one arm...all done...washing the other arm."

It's important to say these things as he's experiencing them so that the words and meaning match. "Here's the washcloth" should be said as you help him pick it up, not when you see it on the side of the tub but he's feeling the running water or picking up a toy boat. Use phrases and short sentences so that he has less information to process and the words more clearly express what's happening. Example: "Books go on the shelf" instead of "Can you help me put the books on the shelf?" Even if he understands the longer sentence, it's less appropriate if he echoes it and is a harder sentence form for him to reuse with other words.

It is very important that your modeled sentences are only a few words longer than what he says spontaneously and appropriately. If he echoes five-word sentences but only creates new ideas in one or two words, you should model two- to three-word phrases. They may need to be short and simple but should be well structured. You don't need to omit words like "a" and "the" or markers like verb tense and possession (is going, went, Daddy's).

As much as possible, avoid questions and direct commands at first and replace them with statements that Lucas can imitate and reuse in similar situations.

For example, say "Time to go to the bathroom," "Gotta go potty" or "Lucas needs to pee" to initiate a bathroom trip, instead of "Do you have to go to the bathroom?" Any of these are more accurate for him to use to ask to go to the bathroom than an echo of "Do you have to go to the bathroom?" If you're mistaken, and he resists or doesn't produce, you can say "No potty now" or "Don't need to go," and try again later. In both cases you've modeled phrases or sentences which are appropriate for him to say spontaneously to tell you he needs, or doesn't need, to use the bathroom.

I've found the carrier phrases "Time to..." and "Let's..." to be good substitutes for some questions and instructions. They minimize the confusing pronouns, give him a model he can use to initiate an activity and are a bit less likely than direct commands to elicit what I call the "automatic No!"

Examples:

"Time to get in line" instead of "You need to get in line now."

"Let's go to the lunch table" instead of "Can you go to the lunch table?"

If he suggests an activity using the carrier phrases you modeled, such as "Time for lunch" and it isn't lunchtime, you can say "Lunch later. First recess, then lunch." Since he is quite invested in the schedule and familiar with the routine, he probably knows this and is actually trying to say "I'm hungry." If you can, model "I'm hungry. Let's have a snack," but be sure you eat too. Any time you say "I," it should be true of you and therefore clear to him that you are speaking of yourself.

If he's obviously enjoying something, you can say "Lucas likes music" or "Mm, that's a good cookie," instead of asking "Do you like it?" which he can't answer yet because he doesn't understand the concept of "Yes" or even say the word "Yes."

Try to omit pronouns much of the time when commenting, especially "I" and "you" and "my" and "your," which are very difficult for echolalic children because their base of reference shifts with each speaker. Use names for now: "Mommy's cooking supper; Dad will tie

Lucas's shoe," "Lucas is playing the piano." When using a schedule, say "Check the schedule" instead of "Check your schedule." "I" can be reintroduced later, followed by "you," but confusion can be minimized if they're eliminated for a while. Also, if you refer to Lucas as "he" too often—for example, telling someone else "He wants to go outside"— you may find him calling himself "he" inappropriately. Referring to himself as "Lucas" is an intermediate step and is an improvement on calling himself "you" or "him."

Some exceptions to the "I" rules

It's okay to use "I" to refer to shared activities when it's appropriate for him to echo it. In fact, this is a good way to help Lucas start using "I" with verbs other than "want." Examples:

1. Both of you are clapping.

    You: I'm clapping.

    Lucas: I'm clapping.

2. He stops to listen to a plane flying overhead.

    You: I hear a plane.

    Lucas: I hear a plane.

    Later, he may hear another plane and say "I hear a plane," which for now may be a delayed echo, but it is also a true, meaningful comment on his experience, spoken in a conventional form. It works.

3. You are playing in the sandbox together. He is digging, so you start digging too and say "I'm digging," and he may echo "I'm digging."

And this is where the hand cue for "I" that you taught with "I want" can help. When you hear Lucas start a sentence with "You" when he means "I"—for example, "You went down the slide?"—touch his fingertips to his chest and he will probably correct to "I went down the slide." The intonation of the corrected statement should sound like a comment, not a question, as he has only practiced "I want..." as statements. Remember, we were careful not to let that sound like a question. But if he does say "I went down the slide?" with a questioning intonation, you just respond with "Went down the slide," which confirms his message without adding to the pronoun confusion or modeling a questioning intonation.

Echolalic children tend to repeat praise also, so try to avoid statements like "Good for you" and "You did it!" Instead, try to praise him by making an enthusiastic comment on the accomplishment. Words like "There, it's done!" "Hurray!" "Yeah!" "Good, all done!" or "Lucas did it!" would be more appropriate if he repeats them. Give him a high five or pat on the back if he enjoys these.

A fill-in-the-blank technique is often helpful when you're trying to avoid questions and still get some information.

Teacher: Lucas went to the playground for recess. Lucas played on the...

Lucas: ...swings.

Just don't overdo it or you may find him stopping his sentences in the middle and expecting you to finish them.

Asking an echolalic child to repeat a sentence by telling him "Say..." often isn't successful because he's likely to repeat the "say" along with the words you want him repeat. I've found this more useful after a base of appropriate communicative language is established and the child is better able to understand what you want him to do. At that point you may want to tell him exactly what to say, as in "Tell Daddy, 'Time for lunch!'" instead of the more confusing, "Tell Daddy to come to lunch."

Helping Lucas learn to play with toys in a meaningful way

is very important. Children learn many concepts about actions, locations, disappearance and reappearance, cause and effect, and other relationships between objects and events through their play. Learning to make appropriate comments about his own activities will help him to connect actions, objects and events with the words that represent them. Here's a sample activity for working on language and play together.

Help Lucas turn the handle on a jack-in-the-box. If possible, guide him at the elbow so he's doing the holding and turning of the handle. Say something like this: "Here's the jack-in-the-box (as you put his hands on it)... Gotta turn the handle (as you help him do so)... Music, it makes music... Oh! Jack popped up! ... Time to push him down...shut the door... Jack's gone down; Jack's in the box... Turning the handle... more music." Be sure to time your words to match his experience.

Book sharing is a good way to model language, but many young autistic children will not sit and listen to a story. I believe this is a language comprehension issue. Word books, which have individual pictures or poster-like scenes with word labels, can be an excellent starting place, especially for someone like Lucas who is hyperlexic and will be drawn to the labels under the pictures. The "reader" can point to and label pictures while modeling noun, verb, adjective and adverb vocabulary, concepts, categories, emotions and sentence structure which will still be accurate and meaningful if Lucas repeats them exactly as he hears them. Examples:

+ This is a tractor. It's a green one.

+ I see some birds. The baby birds are in the nest.

+ This girl looks sad. She is crying.

+ Wow, that's a tall giraffe. It has a long neck.

+ And look, here's a turtle. Turtles move very slowly. They can't go fast.

- This page is all pictures of fruit. Grapes are fruit, oranges are fruit and apples are fruit.

- Here's an outdoor picture. I see water and grass and sky.

If he's not looking where you point, try using his finger to point. He's more likely to look at that. Don't hurry, pause often, and when he's paying attention well, prompt him to add comments, perhaps with a starter phrase like "This is a…" or "The school bus is…" No questions needed.

Some important things to remember in language modeling during play are:

- Say things that match what's happening from the child's point of view.

- Avoid questions and instructions.

- Say things that will still be accurate if echoed by the child.

- Say them as they happen.

- Use short phrases, even if he's echoing whole sentences.

- Don't say exactly the same thing every time. With a Jack-in-the-box, vary from "Oh, Jack popped up" to "Jack came up" to "Here's Jack" and so on.

- Don't talk excessively. Pause and allow him to time to process what you've said and to say something himself.

Making choices

Lucas does not respond reliably to a verbal choice such as "Do you want an apple or a cracker?" He is likely to say "Apple or cracker?" or just "Or cracker?" Repeating both offers, or only the second one, with a questioning intonation is echoing, not answering.

So, omit the question for a while. Just show the two items, moving each one closer to him as you name it: "Cracker...apple...Lucas wants..." leaving a blank for him to fill in. It should sound like a statement, not a question. If he names one and takes it, say "Lucas wants the apple" or "Want some apple!" to confirm his choice as you give it to him. If he says nothing and just reaches for one, say "Apple!" and pause before releasing it. There's a good chance he'll echo it, but if not, just name it one more time and give it to him. Avoid saying "You want an apple" or "Okay, here's your apple," because he may use your words, with the incorrect pronouns, to initiate a spontaneous request later.

Rejecting objects or prohibiting actions

If he pushes away his spinach or resists when his face is being washed, help him push it away or back off and say "No spinach!" or "Don't want spinach!" or "No washing face," modeling what he could say to protest. Sometimes you can accept his refusal, but in other cases you'll need to overrule him by saying something like "Lucas doesn't like face washing (pause, gently squeeze his shoulder or make some other empathic response, then go on)...Lucas's face is dirty... Mommy's gotta wash it."

If someone tries to take his toy, help him pull it back and say "Give it back!" or "Don't take it!" Clap your hands repeatedly and then tell yourself "No clapping" or "Stop" or "Don't," and then immediately stop. Model "Stop!" and "Go" during action games like swinging, spinning or riding in a swivel chair. As you can see, this overlaps with directing actions. The ability to request, protest and direct people verbally can be a big help in avoiding tantrums.

Goal #3: Lucas will respond to the greetings "Hi," "Hello," "Good morning" and "Bye" or "Goodbye" without echoing his own name and will call three familiar people by name in his response.

Another common area of difficulty for echolalic children is greetings.

Because Lucas tends to repeat "Hi, Lucas" when you greet him, try these ideas:

* Just say "Hi" or "Bye" without adding his name.

* If you need to get his attention, say "Lucas" and then, after he glances at you, "Bye." You can repeat the "Bye" and help him wave if necessary, to get a response. For "Hi," he may be more likely to respond if you bridge the gap between you by putting his hand on your face or shoulder to direct his attention, but it is usually easier at first to get a response to "Bye." "Bye" has a clear association; someone leaves. But "Hi" is just a starter for more interaction.

* Encourage people you see regularly to greet him as described above and to say things that will be accurate if echoed, as in the example below.

Mrs. Smith: "Bye" or "See you later" or "See you next Wednesday" (not "Come again soon, Honey" or another farewell that's inappropriate if repeated by the child who's leaving).

Of course, once he learns not to echo his own name in greetings, we want him to start using the other person's name. His mother can model having Lucas say goodbye before Mrs. Smith says it to him.

Mom: Bye, Mrs. Smith (helping Lucas wave).

Lucas: (echoing) Bye, Mrs. Smith.

It might help if his mother moves his hand to touch Mrs. Smith's arm as she models her name. Hyperlexia could help here too. Since Lucas likes, and is able, to read name tags, practicing with a few people wearing, and pointing to, name tags when they greet him could help him learn this social skill. Keep in mind that Hellos and Goodbyes are social behaviors, and some autistic children with greater verbal skills have told me that greetings seem meaningless because no information is exchanged.

Goal #4: Lucas will participate in, or lead, a modified "Simon Says" game with a group of his preschool classmates.

A modified version of "Simon Says"—I call it "Everybody"—provides good practice in taking and giving directions with peers. The leader sits in a chair in front of a row of classmates in chairs. The chairs help to keep everyone anchored in place. The leader says and demonstrates an instruction such as "Everybody stand up" or "Everybody jump" or "Everybody clap." The children in the row of chairs imitate the leader and rotate through turns being the leader. It is easy for adults to prompt children through the actions as they are learning. If Lucas is the leader and isn't initiating an instruction, he may echo an adult prompter or fill in a direction if the adult says "Everybody" with a rising intonation. Children usually all enjoy the game, and are learning to listen to each other, to direct other people and to participate as part of a group.

This combination of goals and activities will help Lucas develop many early functional communication skills in conventional non-echoic forms, including requesting, directing, protesting, commenting, choosing and greeting, while enhancing his meaningful play. But there is still much more to learn, some of which we will address when we meet Seth in the next chapter.

Chapter 6

Echolalia or Not

Seth and Terek

Lucas and Seth illustrate two points along the continuum from echolalia to more conventional conversation. Seth has met most of the goals set for Lucas and will be working on later communication goals associated with echolalia. Seth has the added complication of blindness, but most of his team would say that autism impacts his life and development more significantly than his total lack of vision.

Terek's language development has progressed gradually, with considerable speech and language therapy, but without echolalia. Nevertheless, any or all of his goals may eventually be relevant for the two younger boys who are now progressing through echolalia.

Seth

Seth is a six-year-old boy who is blind as a result of Leber congenital amaurosis and has an autism spectrum diagnosis. He has had early intervention services since infancy and now attends a mainstream kindergarten class with one-to-one assistance from a paraprofessional.

Seth speaks clearly, often in complete sentences, in a combination of immediate and delayed echoes and novel utterances. That is, he sometimes repeats exactly what he just heard in conversation directed to him or overheard from conversations of others in the room or on television, and he sometimes repeats chunks of language he has heard in past similar situations. But he increasingly creates new phrases and sentences from his own ideas. He is fairly proficient in the goals that Lucas was working on, including using the pronoun "I" with "want" and a variety of other verbs, greeting known people by name, playing with a number of familiar problem-solving toys and effectively requesting, directing, protesting and occasionally commenting on his actions.

However, while working with a teacher he often sings loudly, and he may keep repeating "Bitty bitty bee, bitty bee, bitty bee" or recite lines from books and movies. He cannot reliably answer yes/no questions, has difficulty generalizing concepts of physical location (under, behind, at the top) beyond the specific lessons in which he has practiced them, and requires constant adult direction to stay focused on learning tasks.

He certainly talks—almost all the time. As is common with autism, Seth's comprehension tends to be literal. One day, his teacher, Ms. Dylan, was showing him how to peel an orange, and Seth was happily chanting his "bitty bees." Earlier that day Ms. Dylan had done a lesson on emotions and now she saw a teachable moment. "Seth," she said, "you are smiling; your lips are curling up. You are feeling..." and Seth cheerfully replied, "An orange!"

Seth asks the people he meets whether they have squishy or hard toilet seats and smooth or carpeted floors. This information about things he often touches but cannot see is an area of strong personal interest to Seth. He also asks questions when he already knows the answers, answers them himself if his listener won't, and will correct people who deliberately give him a wrong answer. These interactions provide him with opportunities for predictable, and therefore comfortable, conversation. He doesn't yet have the communicative flexibility to converse naturally.

He remembers the specific information he has elicited from many conversational partners, such as their birth dates, ages, toilet seat construction and car brands. He remembers people's names and recognizes voices quickly, and will announce the presence of an occasional consultant visiting his classroom if she just clears her throat nearby. Although Seth is blind, it is difficult to observe him without being discovered.

Seth maneuvers around familiar spaces quite efficiently and quickly becomes comfortable moving around new rooms. Peer interaction is minimal, but he will play the "Everybody" game that Lucas is learning and will tolerate taking turns with a toy if an adult facilitates the interaction. He loves music and can play a dozen songs on the piano by ear.

He has a strong "automatic No!" when asked or told to do things or to shift from one activity to another, especially when he is uncertain that the suggested activity will be comfortable for him. He cannot shift his attention readily and he frequently shrieks loudly when he is expected to stop an activity that he does not feel he has finished. Seth is learning to travel with a cane and will sometimes use it, with remarkable accuracy, to whack an adult helper if he is distressed.

Seth uses "No!" to refuse, protest or prohibit another person's behavior, but he does not use it to deny the accuracy of a question. If given a ball and asked "Is this a shoe?" he might say "Ball," but he would not say "No." If asked, "Is it a ball?" he would probably repeat the end of the question for affirmation, saying "ball," but he essentially never says the word "Yes."

Seth has a variety of verbal and physical behaviors that complicate his learning and he benefits from the predictability of the tactile schedule that his teachers have created for him. Some other helpful accommodations they use include clear expectations, simple explanations, advance notice of coming transitions, minimizing wait times between activities, and assisting him through difficult situations with a calm, supportive "I'll help" attitude. All of these will help decrease the frequency of his "automatic No!" and the number of cane bruises on the shins of his helpers.

Meanwhile, he will be working on goals for answering "yes" or "no," eliminating extraneous jabbering during teaching sessions, learning to work independently on a series of familiar tasks, and guiding himself through hygiene routines and indoor travel with his cane.

Goal #1: When working individually with a teacher, Seth will refrain from singing, reciting from books or movies and jabbering nonsense syllables.

"Chanting" is the name we chose to refer to Seth's sing-songy tendency to echo lines from movies and books, and recite "Bitty bee, bitty bee, bitty bee." Others might call it scripting or chattering or jabbering, but it does need a name. We won't interrupt Seth's use of this delayed echoing and perseveration when he is engaged in free play by himself, but we will sometimes join his activity and model language that goes with his play. For now, the goal is that he won't do the "chanting" while working with an adult. Here is a process for teaching him to inhibit it.

When he echoes lines from movies or books or perseverates on his "bitty bees" during individual work times, tell him "That's chanting." For about three weeks, just do this and redirect him to the tasks you are doing. Don't tell him not to do it, just label it. Ignore it during free play or other situations when you are not directly working with him.

After he has heard his extraneous vocalizations referred to as "chanting" for a few weeks, choose a familiar, directed school task that he can do quickly and easily. Before you start, put out a card with the words "No chanting" brailled on it, touch his hand to it, say "No chanting" and do the activity. Be brief; even just a give him a few quick directions like "Touch your head" and "Knock on the desk" to ensure success. At the end, put his fingers on the braille words again, say "No chanting, good!" and give him a token. Do a few more short tasks, and when he has three tokens, trade them for a reward. Try to run the whole sequence quickly for several days to help him understand the process before expecting it to succeed with longer regular tasks. If he does start chanting, say "Uh-oh, no chanting. Try again," and do a few more quick tasks before giving him the token. If he really can't inhibit the extraneous vocalizing some days, end the activity, pleasantly saying something like "Too much chanting; no more tokens now," and change locations to another activity.

Pay attention to the times the chanting is occurring. You may find that it is sometimes an indication of stress, such as an attempt to drown out teaching that he is not understanding, or anxiety simply because the expectation is new. In these situations, a supportive teacher makes a big difference. Saying something like "It's okay; I'll help" and doing the task yourself for a while can help calm him.

Another possibility is that the "bitty bees" help him relax during alone times, or shut out the noise of the other children playing around him. It could also be, or become, habitual: "I do it here because I did it here yesterday."

When he can reliably complete several learning activities without "chanting," generalize to other people and places who work one-on-one with Seth, then to different contexts such as group activities or walking in the hall. For now, don't worry about times he is alone playing or working independently. When independent work (Goal #3) is well established, that could be the next place to work on inhibiting chanting.

Goal #2: Seth will reliably and accurately answer "yes" or "no" questions referring to characteristics of objects, such as "Is it a...?"

Because we are trying to teach him the concept of "yes," it is better to ask a question that we are sure has a known correct answer rather than "Do you want...?" in which the evidence is fuzzy. If Seth says "Yes," takes the offered item and just drops it, did he really want it? Or was he saying "yes" because he thought that was the "correct" answer? So we will start with "Is it a...?"

To teach him to answer "Is it a...?" it helps to combine it with a sorting activity. Have a YES box and a NO box, with brailled labels attached. Touch and read the labels with him and say "This box is for 'yes' and this box is for 'no.'" It is very important that the items you use for sorting are already well known to Seth.

Hold a ball in his hand, ask "Is it a ball?" Pause briefly and answer "Yes!" and help him put it in the YES container. It is even better if you can let him feel the ball but have another person say "yes" so you don't answer your own question. Do this repeatedly with other balls. After a few samples, he should answer "yes" as an echo, then if you just start the word ("Yyye..."), and then with no prompting.

Next give him a sock, continue to say "Is it a ball?" and model "No!" and put it in the NO container. Repeat by randomly alternating the balls with socks and other objects he knows such as combs and spoons, but don't change the question. Always ask "Is it a ball?" You may need to help for a while by saying "no" or "nnnn..." as you did with "yes," but he should soon start to say "yes" when given a ball and "no" when given any other item. You will end up with a container of balls and a container of non-balls.

When he reliably answers correctly, do the same activity but ask about another familiar item, such as socks ("Is it a sock?") or triangles ("Is it a triangle?"), so the YES box ends up full of socks or triangles and the NO box is a collection of other things. For now, the question names only the item that goes in the YES box ("Is it a triangle?"), so he only needs to focus on "yes" or "no." Then we need to teach him to answer even if the question keeps changing.

Start mixing up the questions by asking "Is it a sock?" and then "Is it a triangle?" for example, being sure that sometimes the answer is "yes" and sometimes it is "no." You will end up with a variety of objects in each box.

When he can answer the mixed questions about objects, ask ones that include attributes such as "Is it a big triangle?" Just be sure you use items and concepts he knows very well; don't try to teach "triangle" or "big" and "yes" in the same activity. You are using labels and attributes he knows very well to teach the concepts of affirmation and negation. Seth can easily discriminate among shapes by touch, and he understands relative sizes, so "big triangle" would work for him. He could not, of course, answer the question "Is it a blue triangle?"

When Seth understands the concept of "yes" to mean "That's right," and "no" to mean "That's wrong," start using them in natural contexts when you know that he knows the information needed to answer. You might ask "Is it raining?" or "Does the ice feel hot?" or even "Do you want...?" if you are quite sure you could predict his choice. You may have to prompt him with "yyye..." or "nnnn..." a few times, but he should quickly generalize his understanding to these other forms of yes/no questions once he has grasped the meaning of "yes" and "no" to affirm or deny a statement.

Goal #3: By himself, Seth will work through a sequence of three familiar tasks, completing each one and transitioning to the next without adult prompting.

Many autistic children and adults have difficulty organizing themselves to play or work independently and spend much of their time either being structured and directed by others or engaging in aimless or perseverative behaviors when given "free time." For these individuals, structured but independent schedules of activities can provide another level of purposeful and enjoyable activity. In addition to providing structure that allows the student to work or play productively with little to no adult involvement for significant lengths of time, it fosters development of a feeling of independence for students who spend most of their time accompanied and directed by adults. Following an activity schedule also can be a precursor to following written directions, doing homework or maintaining focus and productivity in employment. The process can be taught to preschoolers or started with teens and young adults. Children of all ages and a wide range of ability seem to learn it easily and enjoy it.

The process I call "independent work" is based on the work/activity systems of the TEACCH program in North Carolina (Mesibov, Shea and Schopler 2005, pp.43–45). Nearly all the students I've used it with have found it motivating and enjoyable, and a lot of parents and teachers have been pleased to see their children begin to work/play productively and independently for 15 to 60 minutes.

Independent work: The process in general

1. Find a consistently available workspace that is fairly free of distractions and where the student feels comfortable. You will soon be able to transfer it to many settings. Non-speaking children have often done familiar independent work in regular education classrooms while their classmates worked on different tasks.

2. Select containers for the activities. A three-drawer plastic chest, as used in this description, is often a good choice, but baskets and boxes have also worked well, or folders for students doing paper-and-pencil activities. Be sure the containers will hold the items you plan to use even after they are assembled. For example, if you are using large puzzles, be sure they can be put away without having to stand them on end in the drawer. The completed work should stay done when the child replaces it in the container. It should not fall apart.

3. Select initial activities to put in the drawers, knowing you can add others later. These should be things the student can already do easily. For children at early developmental stages, these are often puzzles, shape sorters, matching/lotto boards that can be Velcroed so the small pieces don't fall off, sorting activities or simple assembly toys.

   As much as possible, older students, even if at early developmental levels, should be provided with tasks and materials that are reasonably age-appropriate. For example, sorting tasks might involve silverware, coins, small hardware items or jewelry parts (if you are certain they won't go in the student's mouth) and assembly might be flashlights or plumbing parts.

   If the student does not have any activities he or she can do without help, you will need to establish some first, *not* within the independent schedule procedure. When you want to add new activities, it may also be necessary to pre-teach them. An activity should not be included in the independent schedule until the student knows exactly how to do it. Seth could start with a shape sorter, nesting cups and a 12-piece puzzle. *Tasks Galore* (Eckenrode, Fennell and Hearsey 2003) provides many ideas for independent work tasks.

4. Make a set of symbols, one for each of the three drawers (Examples: circle, square, triangle, 1-2-3). Because Seth is learning braille, his symbols will be the braille letters A, B and C made out of beads embedded into thick cardboard. Use Velcro to mount one symbol on the front of each of the drawers so that you have, for example, a drawer A and a B and a C. Provide a container to drop the symbols into when each task is completed.

5. You have set the stage; there are three drawers, each marked with a symbol and each containing a toy or task you know the student can do without help and that has a distinct end. Reading a book would not be a good choice for independent work because there is no clear evidence that it is completed. You won't know if he did it, and unless he reliably reads through from beginning to end, the child may not know when to stop. Likewise, drawing pictures or writing stories, though wonderful activities, don't have obvious ending points.

Be sure that when you put the materials in the drawer, they are unassembled. The student is learning to find a task that needs to be done, do it and put it away completed, so we don't want him to take it apart before or after doing it. If there are multiple pieces, it helps to have them in a small container in the drawer so the student can take them out easily.

6. Provide whatever introductory explanation is needed or helpful for your particular student. For some, this means say nothing and just visually direct him to the drawers, then assist and demonstrate the expected behaviors. For Seth it might be something like: "It's

time to do independent work. I will help while you are learning but I won't talk. You can learn to do these things alone."

Regardless of the introduction, the help you give during the process should be nonverbal and as minimal as possible. The idea is that eventually you won't be there at all, so try very hard not to introduce verbal cues that the student on the autism spectrum is likely to see as an essential part of the process. An autistic child will often wait for you to say "What's next?" or "What should you be doing?" even when he knows, just because he thinks it is a required part of the learned routine. So try very hard not to talk.

7. Assist him through the process of opening the first drawer, putting the contents on his workspace, doing the task, replacing the completed item in the drawer, closing it, pulling off the symbol and putting it in the provided container and repeating the process with the next drawer. A slotted container for the symbols from completed drawers is often appealing to the child, but an open box will do. If necessary, use gentle physical prompts, points and gestures or a tap on the item that needs attention. Even start the task yourself to demonstrate if necessary, but *don't talk*. For nonverbal prompting, do as much as necessary to get through the process smoothly and without long delays, but as little as you can get away with, and always be trying to reduce it. If you must prompt at beginnings and ends of tasks, try to move away while the student works on the familiar task. Remember, your goal is to not be there at all. Typically, the last part an autistic child does without prompting is opening the next drawer after putting away a completed activity.

In a prominent location, perhaps at the bottom front of the third drawer, attach a small card that says "all done," in braille for Seth. Teach him to pull it off, give it to you and announce that he has finished the work. Later, expect him to come find you to report that he has completed the independent work.

Goal #4: Seth will independently complete his hand-washing routine and travel to two familiar places in the school without adult assistance or prompting.

Independence in routines

For things you want Seth to do alone (following the schedule, toileting, hand washing), prompt him with nonverbal cues and simple scripts like "Water on...hands in the water...need soap...rub, rub, rub...rinse... need a towel." Move him smoothly through the actions, not rushing but without delays, saying the script *as* you do the actions. Then start leaving out words and fading physical prompts until he is doing it alone. Think of it as teaching him words that he can say to himself to remind him of the steps. If he gets distracted, just add gentle physical assistance. Avoid questions and directives when you want independence. Children on the autism spectrum are very prone to waiting for your questions even when they know what to do; they seem to think it is a necessary part of the routine. I especially try to avoid "What should you do next?"

On the playground, Seth used to resist letting his feet leave the ground but now he's using a few different pieces of equipment. Modeling language to match his use of new equipment may help him become competent more quickly. Don't look for simpler vocabulary for the names of things. Call the bars on the climbing equipment vertical, horizontal and diagonal. He will quickly learn these terms. These terms and words like "right" and "left" are used early and frequently in orientation and mobility instruction for visually impaired children. Say things like "Hands on the vertical bars...feet on the horizontal bars...hands slide down...step down...step down...here's the mulch!" as you help him. This gives him reminders he can memorize and use to prompt himself, like the hand washing described above. Be vigilant; don't expect common sense in safety.

To help him leave the slide without a meltdown, give a measurable warning like "One more up, one more down, then the swing." When he is at the top, say "One more down, then the swing." Then be prepared to meet him at the bottom of the slide, saying "All done with the slide. Time to swing," and start him moving toward the swing even though he may be squawking a bit.

To help him find his way from the school bus to his classroom, model language that matches his movements as he walks, encounters objects and sweeps his cane side to side:

> "Straight along the sidewalk...here's the school door" (as he finds it with his hand or cane) "...it's open" (as he pulls it open) "...in the hall; gotta turn right..." (sweep, sweep, sweep) "...here's the wall..." (sweep, sweep) "...it's a doorway...Mr. Johnson's room..." (sweep, sweep, sweep) "...here's a doorway...Mrs. Allen's room...found the threshold...right turn...gotta find the hooks..."

Each thing you say to him would be a comment on what he is experiencing, as he hits it with his cane (which you may be helping him sweep from side to side as you model this) or a comment on what comes next. All should be said as if he were talking to himself, *not* as questions or instructions. The idea is to give him a script to memorize and say to himself, aloud at first and later silently, to help him travel independently. Try to say it the same way each time (write it down), and after a few times, pause and let him fill in parts until he can do it alone.

Some other thoughts for Seth

Understanding concepts of location (on, between, top)

Concepts of location require recognizing the shifting, temporary relationship between objects; paper and book keep the same names, but the paper can be on, in or under the book. For autistic children who are relying heavily on memory, it is hard to keep track of the salient features.

Seth does well in practice sessions, but is still confused by words like between, beside and top when they are used in new situations.

Teach the same concept in varied situations and he will eventually make the connection. For example, the "top" of a paper is not the same as the top of his head or a bookcase or the slide or the family car, and the top of the paper is not the same as the top paper in a pile. With enough examples he will deduce the rule that top means the highest part of whatever we are talking about.

When teaching, model more often than you test. For example, as he touches the top of the bookcase, either spontaneously or when you physically prompt him, say "This is the top of the bookcase." Don't ask him to "find the top" independently until you are pretty sure he knows, because his errors will further confuse him. Concepts of location and direction (right, left, straight) are very important orientation information for blind children, and Seth has been hearing them from his orientation and mobility instructors for a long time.

Other bits

For now, say things in the order they will happen to avoid confusion. "First circle time, then snack" rather than "Snack is after circle time" or "Before snack we have circle time." Although we do want him to understand these language forms, for now it will be easier for him to process a sequence of events mentioned in the order they will occur. Less confusion equals fewer meltdowns.

Don't say "No thank you!" if you mean "Don't do that!" "Thank you" is likely to be confusing anyway and this will make it more so.

Avoid, or specifically teach, non-literal expressions like "Give me your ears," to which Seth may shriek, "No, I need my ears!" Even "Pay attention" may be confusing, since paying is something you do with money in a store.

As these and other goals are met, Seth's communication will become more like Terek's, or perhaps like Mia's in Chapter 8.

Terek

Terek is navigating the often troubled waters of middle school. He has never been significantly echolalic and has language that is adequate for daily-life activities. Many of his communication behaviors will probably be true for Lucas and Seth when they are a bit older and could also impact the children in the advanced language group.

Middle school can be a daunting chapter in any child's life. Nor is it easy for the parents and teachers shepherding these young adolescents. For Terek, who is autistic and has delays in language and academic development, it is especially taxing.

He is 12 ("and a half!") years old and in seventh grade. Terek has an educational plan that includes time in mainstream and resource classrooms. A paraprofessional accompanies him to his regular education classes and helps him with the schoolwork. He is strong in spelling, geography and factual information that can be memorized. His oral reading is more monotone than expressive, but he can decode words well. His comprehension, especially when reading fiction, is much weaker than his oral reading. Math is not a strength and word problems are especially difficult for Terek. Most of his math and language arts work is done in the resource room at approximately a fourth-grade level. He attends mainstream classes in science, computer, art, music and physical education with some assistance and modifications. Terek sometimes goes "elsewhere" in his mind when a class is difficult for him, and may giggle, laugh aloud or blurt out a comment related to his thoughts. He often appears to be replaying video games in his mind.

His teachers recognize that he needs academic support but describe him as being prompt-dependent, meaning that he seems not to listen to group directions and then waits for them to come and help him start his work. They say he needs this jump-start from them even for familiar tasks that he can do easily. And sometimes they are frustrated by Terek's apparent inattention while they are helping him. His science teacher, standing by Terek's desk, said, "Come on, Terek, pay attention. I'm bending over backwards to try to help you!"—to which literal

Terek replied, "No, you're not. You're standing up straight." Much of his inattention is the result, not the cause, of his weak comprehension.

Terek tends to talk in lengthy monologues about his favorite topics, currently car brands and models, and he is rarely able to maintain a conversation on topics introduced by others. He resists letting others break into his monologues to add information or ask questions. Terek spends much of his time alone, interacting only occasionally with his peers. He shows some stereotypical behaviors such as mild rocking, hand flapping down by his sides and pacing. These are minimal in classes but much more obvious when he is moving about the school.

Terek has developed an intense interest in a girl, Arielle, at his school, saying that he loves her and is going to marry her. She is reportedly a friendly young lady who has interacted nicely with Terek but does not want to be his girlfriend and is upset by his excessive attention. A few months ago, Terek was making similar comments about a favorite teacher.

Especially troubling is his tendency to lash out verbally, and sometimes physically, when he is confused, stressed or angry. He shouts threats at teachers or other students and will hit, kick or push people if he feels cornered. Despite being generally a bit lethargic and slow to respond, Terek reacts strenuously to unexpected noise or touch. These sensory "assaults" are often the cause of his outbursts.

Terek will have four specific goals for decreasing his verbal aggression, conversing on a topic for several turns, interacting more appropriately with Arielle and other peers, and starting schoolwork more independently. Social narratives and incentive plans will figure strongly in his intervention plans, for these goals and for some of the other issues mentioned.

Social narratives, the offspring of Carol Gray's Social Stories™ (Gray 2010), are:

• individualized stories or explanations, presented in visual and spoken form

• written by parents and teachers at the child's level of understanding

♦ to explain social situations and describe appropriate words and actions to use

♦ to help autistic students regulate behavior, communicate better, interact with peers, and live more comfortably and cooperatively.

Incentive plans focus on a specific issue that the child is capable of changing, use concrete language to describe a behavior that is observable and objective, and provide a strong enough reward to motivate the child to change.

Goal #1: Terek will significantly decrease his use of verbal threats and eliminate physical aggression. With assistance, he will begin to state the problem when he is upset.

When he is upset, because someone bumped into him, or too many kids are scraping their chairs on the floor, Terek is likely to slam his fist on his desk and yell something like "You're mean! I'm gonna kick you for that!" or "Stop that stupid noise or I will smash you all!" He rarely even leaves his seat after these alarming shouts, but if the teacher and assistant hurry over to admonish or calm him, they might get hit or pushed. In both cases, Terek is responding with anger and aggression because he feels threatened. Initially, the bump or noise startled and stressed him and then the looming teachers, even if intending to help, appeared to be a threat. He might recover more quickly if his teachers kept their distance, assured him that they would address the problem and reminded his classmates that bumps and noises upset Terek. However, even if we believe that Terek is responding from fear, his words and behaviors scream "Aggression!" and are not acceptable at school.

To help Terek learn to inhibit these outbursts, I would combine a social narrative, to explain the situation to Terek, with an incentive plan, to motivate him. Both would be put in writing and implemented only after he understood and agreed with them. It might go like this:

Being safe at school

Because it is very important for everyone in every school to feel safe and comfortable during their school day, Terek needs to learn to stop saying some things and doing some actions.

Some things that are never okay to *do* at school include:

+ hit, kick, grab or bite people

+ push things off the table

+ shake your fist at people.

Some things that are never okay to *say* at school include:

+ Words, phrases or sentences about hurting someone, such as "I'm gonna...hit, kill, clobber, smash..." someone.

Everyone gets upset sometimes. Some things that are okay to do when you are upset at school include:

+ go to the beanbag chair

+ ask to get a drink of water

+ ask to go out for some air

+ ask for a break to read favorite magazines

+ sigh, stomp, shake your head and walk away

+ put your head down on your desk.

Some things that are okay to say when you are upset at school include:

- Please don't bump me!

- I am upset because...

- I don't like that noise!

- That hurts my ears!

- It's not fair that...

Because it will be hard for Terek to change some of the "never okay" things that he might say or do when he is upset, we will offer rewards for not using these actions and words.

For every 30 minutes that passes without any of the "never okay" language or behavior happening, Terek will earn two points. If the "not okay" things happen, the time will start over. The points Terek earns will be added up and reported to Terek's parents who will provide a menu of rewards he can earn. Different rewards will have different prices, so Terek can spend points for a small reward or save them up for a larger one.

This is a sample; clearly some schools would have different options for acceptable responses when he is upset, and rewards would often be given at school instead of at home. Also, other specific examples could be added to the "never okay" list as they occur. Important features of the plan include:

- brief mention of the reason why a change is needed

- specific expectations of what to change

- what to do instead

- an incentive for trying to comply with the new expectations.

Goal #2: (a) Terek will converse with one other person, on a topic not chosen by him, until each person has had three conversational turns.

(b) When speaking on one of his favorite topics, Terek will tolerate another person adding to the conversation.

Develop a social narrative to use in speech/language therapy or individual instruction or home practice. Here is a sample:

Staying on the topic

In a conversation, people take turns talking. The topic of a conversation is the thing the people are talking about. If they are talking about trains, the topic is trains. If they are talking about swimming and suntan lotion and playing in the sand, the topic is the beach. If they are talking about pie and cake and pudding, the topic is... (Terek fills in dessert, sweets, etc.).

When two people have a conversation, both people do some of the talking. They usually keep talking about the same topic for several turns. We will practice having conversations where each of us takes three turns saying something about a topic. We will try to stay on the topic and not talk about other things.

We will choose the topic by turning over one of these cards. I will go first. If the card says "Birds," I need to say something about birds. I might say "Some birds built a nest on my porch." Then it is your turn. You need to say something about birds. You might say "What kind of birds were they?" or "Maybe they will lay eggs in the nest." You can tell me something or ask a question, but it needs to be about birds, because birds are the topic of this conversation.

When we start, we will each have three plastic tokens. Each time we say something about birds we can put a token in this bowl. When all the tokens are in the bowl, we can keep talking about birds if we want or one of us can say "Let's change the topic" and choose another card from the pile.

After we have practiced with five topic cards, you can choose any topic you want to talk about, but we will still take turns saying things.

This last piece may be the hardest for Terek, because he will probably choose a topic for which he wants to do all the talking. This expectation involves shifting his monologues to be more like a conversation. You may need to maintain the three tokens to track turns and perhaps offer an incentive such as a special snack or ten minutes' computer time when the practice session is done.

Goal #3: Terek will interact with peers in ways that are not viewed as stalking or harassment.

This is particularly an issue with one female classmate right now, so start with a social narrative to help with that.

Talking to Arielle

Arielle is a nice girl. You like her a lot. Seventh graders do not get married and do not say "I love you" at school. Here are some things you can say to Arielle:

• Hi, Arielle! I'm happy to see you!

• Have a nice weekend.

• I went camping last weekend.

• Did you finish the math homework?

Keep adding to the list to give him a variety of quick conversation starters. Encourage conversation practice with a variety of peers. He may not be able to keep the conversation going, so practicing topics of interest to peers is an important part of Goal #2.

If necessary, you can also make a list of things *not* to say and even pay him with a reward system for inhibiting those things. This would be familiar to Terek from his work on verbal aggression (Goal #1).

> **Goal #4**: (a) Without being prompted, Terek will complete a sequence of three independent work tasks and return them to the teacher.
>
> (b) When given familiar schoolwork during a class, Terek will initiate and complete it without individual prompting from his teacher.
>
> (c) When told a task might be challenging but encouraged to attempt it, Terek will take some pre-planned initial steps before requesting help.

(a) Teach Terek to do a sequence of familiar papers independently. He will find them in the left pocket of a folder, do them and put them in the pocket on the right. He should then give you the folder and tell you that he is done. Explain to Terek that he can ask for help if needed, but this is independent work and you expect that he will be able to do it himself and that you won't be talking to him while he works. Use two or three short papers that you know he can do independently without instruction. The goal is for him to remain focused on his work and transition himself from one paper to the next and, upon completion, report to you that he is finished. If he does need prompting for a while, try to do it nonverbally, by walking by and pleasantly tapping a paper or handing him his pencil.

(b) Make a list with Terek of routine class work you know he can do by himself. This might more often be resource-room vocabulary and math rather than seventh-grade tasks. Tell him you know he can do it because it is just like other work he has done. It is almost like independent work. His job is to start it and you will check in to see how he is doing.

(c) If you are not sure he can do the work independently, ask him to put his name on the paper, read the directions, which you have highlighted, and try to start the work. Help quite promptly if he is struggling because he will be upset about starting over, and you want him to trust the system. This will also be mostly resource-room work but might include starting a science lab with a seventh-grade partner or a slightly new computer task by himself.

You might develop a coding system with Terek where you tell him, for example, "This is type 2 work" and he knows that means:

Type 1 work: You won't need help.

Type 2 work: You probably won't need help.

Type 3 work: You might need help but try it yourself first.

In all cases, help is available if needed, but he becomes more responsible for not just assuming someone needs to be with him. It would be a good idea to have all this in writing for his reference and yours.

Terek has several goals that involve incentive plans and he would probably benefit from a coordinated token economy to support these and other goals around academics, life skills and behavior. Incentive plans and token economy will be described in more detail in Part III.

Chapter 7

Atypical Language: Expanded

As they learn to talk, many autistic children echo whole chunks of the language of other people. They may be echoing complete sentences they have heard and associated with the current situation without understanding how the words and intonation patterns should vary with the speaker's role in the conversation. Because they are using strong memories and verbal imitation skills without good understanding of language, they are often saying the sentences adults have said to them instead of clearly expressing their own intended meaning.

This leads to children saying things like:

+ "Do you want some more?" or "He wants another one" or "Want some juice?" when asking for things.

+ "Try it! It's delicious!" while pushing away an unwanted food.

+ "Are you okay?" or "Are you hurt?" or "You're okay" when they fall.

+ "Do you need help?" or "Open it for you?" to ask for help.

+ "Swing or slide?" or perhaps "Or slide" in response to "Do you want to swing or slide?"

+ "Say goodbye Doctor!" to mean "Get me out of here!"

Many of these echoes sound like questions because the children are repeating things they hear, and adults ask children a lot of questions.

Echolalia is very atypical expressive language, but it is fairly common among children on the autism spectrum, especially when blindness and autism intersect. Children who echo use their strong memories, and often well-articulated speech, to take their conversational turns and to communicate intentionally. However, their listeners are required to interpret the meaning. Also, the echoes don't provide a solid language basis for learning.

Typically developing young children beginning to talk do imitate adult speech, but in smaller chunks of key words and phrases. When you ask a toddler if she wants a cookie, she may say "cookie" or "want cookie" and may use those same words later to ask for another cookie, but she won't say "You want cookie?" Her request is immature, but conversationally appropriate. Non-echolalic children may misuse "me" for "I," as in "Me want some," but are very unlikely to refer to themselves as "you" or "he" or "she" as an echoing child would.

Some children who echo talk a lot; some are more passive and speak infrequently. Their language is often based on association. Something reminds them of past events, and they repeat language they heard in that situation. For example, Sahara hears her sister, Tori, telling her friend about the hurricane they experienced on their last vacation. Although it is now warm and sunny, Sahara exclaims, "It is raining very hard! Close the windows!" Another child might squeal "Say goodbye Doctor!" even in non-medical situations to signal a need to escape.

Many echo speech clearly, sometimes with the intonation pattern and accent of the original speaker. Others sound mumbly and garbled, but their intelligibility often improves spontaneously as more meaningful language develops.

Children who echo language need to learn to express basic functions of requesting, directing, choosing, greeting, commenting, protesting, rejecting and answering or asking questions in a conventional form so they will be better understood. Language supports learning and literacy, and they need more effective communication for education and social interaction.

Some autistic children progress through a phase of echoing and gradually develop more conventional communication; others stay echoic into adulthood. Many need help to move beyond this confusing state of communication. "Wait and see if it goes away" may not be a wise approach.

Echolalia: Lucas and Seth

Lucas attempts to request, direct, choose, reject and protest, and respond verbally, but with echoes instead of standard language. Like many children on the autism spectrum, he is less likely to initiate comments or greetings, although he may respond with a turn-taking echo of "Hi, Lucas" when someone greets him. All the early communicative functions are important and are usually learned and used by typically developing toddlers through play and interaction. Pronouns are ubiquitous and essential in conversation.

Because we must teach meaning, not just word order, we need a context. Play and the activities of daily living work well for Lucas's goals, especially since he also needs to develop meaningful play to replace his repetitive actions with toys. Most of his communication work takes place in natural contexts and should generalize to similar situations readily. As he accomplishes the goals set in Chapter 5, Lucas will need to address some of the communication goals written for Seth in Chapter 6.

Echolalia leaves a legacy. It is not just a peculiar way of talking but a reflection of how the child is thinking. Continued problems with language and learning, social interaction and behavior should be expected.

Seth, having accomplished the goals set for Lucas, still has communication problems associated with echolalia, such as inability to answer yes/no questions, excessive vocalizing in place of verbal interaction, and prompt dependency in areas where he should be more independent. Some of these are also difficult for autistic children who have not been echolalic.

Direct structured practice will help Seth learn the concept of "yes" and its juxtaposition to "no" in answers to questions beginning with "Is it a...?" In most cases, I have seen children who echo quickly generalize to other yes/no questions such as "Are you (verb)ing?" or "Do you want...?" once they grasp the concepts of yes/no answers. In addition to the yes/no confusion, children who echo language may have trouble with concepts of mental activity. They may be confused by "I don't know," "How do you know?" and "Maybe."

I approach the inhibition of Seth's chanting directly with reinforcement to give him some incentive for stopping a behavior that has become somewhat automatic for him. If we expect him to comply, he must first understand the expectation, so we label the behavior for a while before starting to reinforce him for inhibiting it. This inhibition may not generalize readily from the setting in which he learned it. Seth will probably need practice in multiple situations, but he is learning the instruction and expected behavior. With reinforcement and accommodations such as an alternative activity, a chew toy, fidget item or a teacher-directed activity, Seth can learn to inhibit chanting in other places.

Unlike the pre-symbolic children, Seth can, and does, talk. I recommended nonverbal prompting for helping Rebecca complete familiar routines, but for Seth I would model scripts he can use to prompt himself. His verbal scripts for travel are like teaching him to talk to himself and direct himself through an activity. Learning to think and use self-talk about his walking routes will be very important to Seth's independent mobility with his cane.

Children who have been echolalic, and some on the autism spectrum with no echolalia, tend to have strong memories and rote skills and may be hyperlexic (spontaneous early readers with comprehension difficulties). Blind children with autism and echolalia often learn braille easily and also have comprehension issues.

...or not: Terek

When the major differences of echolalic language have been resolved, these children are still on the autism spectrum and will face additional struggles with communication and interaction. These may be much like the difficulties of moderately verbal autistic children who have been acquiring language—probably with the help of speech/language therapy—without the complications of echolalia.

Remember, Terek does not have a history of significant echolalia, but he does have communication issues which are typical of autism spectrum disorders and these will likely be shared by Lucas and Seth as they progress beyond echolalia.

Terek has communication skills that are adequate for general life activities. He can request, direct, comment, greet, answer and ask questions. He has learned these through speech/language therapy, assistance from his parents, his education and life experiences, without the additional confusion of having been echolalic. Likewise, he was not hyperlexic, but he did learn to decode printed words fairly readily at school. However, his more limited reading comprehension and cognitive flexibility interfere with completing math word problems, understanding fiction and learning abstract information. He lacks the cognitive and communicative facility to converse easily, to interpret different types of personal relationships, or to deal calmly with stress or misunderstandings. His comprehension difficulties make it difficult for Terek to remain attentive in class.

Terek's goals relate to interactions at school. Communication and behavior intersect here a lot. Learning to explain what is bothering him and not automatically default to threats will be important at school and vital in employment. He needs to learn how to interact with girls as peers and friends before worrying about them as dates. To acquire friends, he needs to modify his monologues and at least "appear" interested in what others have to say.

Social narratives, direct practice and incentive plans figure strongly in his treatment plan.

Other skills to teach

The goals of Chapters 5 and 6 are not the only difficulties the children in this group face, and do not address their likely strengths. For example, echolalia often goes with good articulation, or it improves with language work, so clarity of speech is not often an issue. Prodigious memory leads to good mastery of factual information, and hyperlexia suggests good academic strength in the early grades. Certainly, the fact that these children are talking opens many avenues for communication intervention, and their memory and knowledge of letters and numbers are an advantage in the early elementary grades.

But autism was previously known as, and continues to be, a "pervasive" developmental disorder. It affects many aspects of development and, despite progress, the disorder persists over time. The language comprehension difficulties that reliably accompany echolalia and hyperlexia become more obvious as a child progresses through school and a good memory becomes insufficient for reasoning about more abstract concepts.

Whether or not they have been echolalic, children and teens on the autism spectrum often have issues with other aspects of speech and language learning. Some of these are also addressed in speech/language therapy for children with delays and disorders not related to autism, and speech/language pathologists and teachers have many ways of addressing them. I will just add a few thoughts about these language problems in relation to ASD.

Applying he/she pronouns to the correct genders

Children with language delays and learning disorders sometimes use object pronouns in place of subject pronouns, as in "Him has a boat" or "Her hit me!" But they are unlikely to be confused about which people go with female or male pronouns, as are some autistic children who might say "He took my book" when the culprit was a girl. This pronoun confusion can often be corrected and practiced with a sorting task.

Using individual pictures of boys and girls, ideally the child's classmates so you can also work on social awareness of real people, sort them into two piles indicated by cards that read "He is a boy" and "She is a girl." Help the child sort the photos, as you name each child and use the correct pronoun to label the child's gender. Say "This is Emily. She is a girl," or "This is Harry. He is a boy." It is okay if you have to say all the words and put the pictures in the correct piles at first and the student just watches. You are demonstrating the connections among a girl picture, the name of a girl, the pronoun "she" and the noun "girl." You are doing the same for the boys, of course. Your student is hearing "she" and "girl" or "he" and "boy" used together repeatedly.

As soon as possible, while maintaining essentially errorless learning, help the student take over the process. Guide him to place the photo in the correct pile as you say the two sentences, then start to leave the second sentence incomplete, such as "This is Harry. He is..." and the child might add "a boy." If not, point to the words on the card labeling the pile and he may read "a boy." Keep leaving off words at the end until the child is reciting both sentences independently and sorting accurately by gender. If the student has difficulty remembering the names of the pictured children, write them on the photos and, if necessary, point to the printed name as you say "This is..." You may need to do the same activity with adults and the labels "man" and "woman."

Expand to object and possessive pronouns and generalize to other situations. Use activities like pointing out children on the playground or in pictures or videos and saying "Look at her. What is she doing?" or "He's getting his coat. That blue coat is his." The plural pronouns "we, us, our, they, them, their" may need some attention too. But with autism and echolalia, the confusion of "I, me, my" with "you, your" is the most significant pronoun conundrum.

Answering "wh" questions (what, who, where, why)

The whole idea of answering a question instead of repeating it can be a problem, and then there is the difficulty of sorting the questions from each other. To start, be sure the child knows the answer before you begin to ask questions. Don't try to teach new information and the process of answering at the same time. For what/who questions, practice just naming pictures of objects or people until the child is accustomed to naming the pictures as you hold them up. Then announce "Question time" and start slipping in the question "What (or who) is this?" as you show the picture. Then do the same with "What is...doing?" "Where is...?" and "What color is it?"

If necessary, model by asking a third person to answer and then have the child take turns by answering a question of the same type just demonstrated by the helper. After several question types are familiar, start mixing them together in a practice session so that "Question time" requires shifting easily among the different types of questions.

Keep in mind that the child may not fully understand the questions and may sometimes answer a question different from the one you asked. Probably, he will revert to the answer for a similar question he understands better. If he has learned to answer "How old are you?" he may say "Four years old," when you have actually asked "How are you?" If you ask "What color is the jacket?" he may say "blue," but if you say "What color is it?" as you point to the jacket, he may say "jacket." If you follow up with "But what color is it?" he will probably tell you "blue." He knew the answer but misinterpreted the question. Visual cues can help while he is learning. For example, you could show a small card with swatches of color when you ask "What color is it?"

For more advanced questions like "Why?" "How?" and "How are these the same/different?" you may need to start by repeatedly modeling a formulaic answer such as "...and...are the same because they both..."

Sometimes you need to know answers before the child understands how to respond to questions. While he is learning, you can sometimes get information using the cloze technique. This just means filling in the blank. You say "Lunch is pizza or chicken. Micah wants..." and he may fill in his choice even if he could not have answered the question "Do you want pizza or chicken for lunch?"

Asking true questions

Although children who echo often use question sentence structure accurately because they have memorized it, and often speak in question forms, they may not ask questions to obtain information.

Try just reversing roles from your practice with answering questions. The child has the pictures, perhaps while sitting in your chair, and says what you said. If he can't remember which question to ask, write them out on cue cards, point to the one he needs and let him read it. Later, have him practice asking about information he really doesn't know, such as unfamiliar people, objects and actions. Use the verb "ask" frequently so child associates it with questioning.

Reading comprehension

Although they may be very skilled at decoding words and able to read aloud easily from texts written for significantly older students, children on the autism spectrum, especially those who have been hyperlexic, very commonly have difficulty with reading comprehension.

Hyperlexia is the combination of early strong, untaught decoding and weak comprehension. It may appear to be a gift or strength in preschool and early elementary grades, when other children are busy learning the decoding aspects of reading. But pay attention to whether the young child who reads well can answer questions, retell the story from just the pictures or talk about the story in relation to his life and experiences.

Children who learn to read spontaneously as toddlers or preschoolers often have difficulty understanding stories they read or hear. One three-year-old I knew could read easily, even if the words were upside down or in a mirror image. But when asked to use only the pictures to retell a story he had read and heard, he refused to try, saying "I can't remember all the words!" Often, if you ask a child with hyperlexia to retell a picture book story as you put your hand over the words, he will try to push away your hand and re-read the story because he didn't understand the gist of the story.

As the child gets into more abstract and complex written text around grade three or four, comprehension problems become more obvious. Sometimes parents are the first to recognize that their child is struggling because of the extensive help needed to complete homework.

When reading with a child who has comprehension difficulty, practice retelling the story with him, paraphrasing and pausing to leave blanks for him to fill in, such as "Jack was crying because..." If he can't do it, fill in the answer for him, as in "Jack was crying because he scraped his knee." After the retelling, review, ask some questions, but also just state information, especially when going beyond the factual information to the why/because/how and emotions. Talk about the title and how it relates to the story, and then summarize the main idea at the end. Don't assume he is making those connections.

Encourage services from reading and speech/language specialists to work on figurative language such as idioms and metaphors, pronoun reference (When it says "his ball," whose ball is it?), words with multiple meanings and abstract vocabulary. Idioms, metaphors and other non-literal language will interfere with understanding text as well as speech. Craig, reading at a third-grade level, did not understand what "looking after other people's children" meant, even though his mother provided day care in their home.

Use the strategies the reading specialists recommend for developing reading comprehension. But recognize that much of the difficulty for autistic children comes from not understanding relationships among people, how thoughts differ and how opinions influence action. Also, they may not have the knowledge of life and the world that supports reading comprehension.

Decoding is a mechanical skill that can be mastered and used in all reading. Comprehension is more complicated and complex but is necessary to gain the learning and enrichment that reading provides.

Interpreting figurative language

This is a long-term project. Around third grade, children are taught about idioms and learn the meaning of many familiar ones. Children who struggle with idioms often work on them more intensely in speech/language therapy. Some autistic children become interested in idioms and metaphors, study them on their own and enjoy using them. But it can be an endless job. Learning the actual meaning of "It's raining cats and dogs" or "Get on the ball" does not mean an autistic child will later understand "She's juggling a lot of plates" or "He was the last adult in the room." It does not even guarantee that he will recognize that these are figurative statements rather than literal descriptions. Teach students to anticipate figurative language and to ask about sentences that seem questionable.

Expect to be explaining figurative meanings, and when possible the rationale behind them, for a long time, as in "Well, she's not really juggling plates, but if she was, she would be having to pay attention to a lot of plates at the same time so she wouldn't drop any of them. So 'juggling a lot of plates' means trying to do a lot of things at the same time."

Considering suggestions or instructions
without automatically saying "No!"

With autism, transitions and shifts of attention are difficult, surprises are generally unwelcome, and predictability and sameness are comforting. So it is not surprising that "No!" is a common response to instructions or suggestions that involve a change of focus or activity. Since this resistance is often immediate and reflexive, I refer to it as the "automatic No!" At times it seems almost like a startle response. View it as a defensive reaction that may or may not signal a solid refusal. Try to interpret and accept it as if the child is saying "Wait a minute, what!?" instead of "No!"

The "automatic No!" often leads to missed opportunities when a child says "no" to something he would have enjoyed. It initiates power struggles when an adult must insist that the child complies, and it interferes with new learning.

I believe it is best to avoid insisting on an immediate response from an autistic child when a change is required. Many people have learned that an advance warning such as "Two minutes until..." can be very helpful. Sometimes providing an announcement of, and exposure to, a coming expectation, without any pressure to conform right now, can smooth the transition. Here are three examples:

- Introducing a new expectation during an individual instruction session: "Here is a game (as you just show the game box) we will look at later." Set it aside and do a familiar activity.

  Later: "Let's look at this game" (as you take out pieces, handle them together and put them back, or perhaps set them up for the start of the game).

  You may need to help or even take the turns for both of you the first time you play the game. If losing is a serious issue for the child, see Goal #2 for Mia in Chapter 8.

- "I'm going to the library at two o'clock. You can come if you want" or "You need to come with me."

  "It's one thirty now. I'm going to the library at two o'clock. You can come if you want/need to come." (Put out his coat and library books.)

  "It's two o'clock. Let's go to the library" as you hand him his coat.

- "Ben will be joining us for speech therapy next week. Here is a picture of him with your favorite game. He will bring that game to play with us." Keep the picture in sight, mention it a few times and maybe even put Ben's picture on the therapy session schedule the day he is coming.

Of course, including new activities on a visual schedule is nearly always a good idea.

Making eye contact during interactions

Limited eye contact is a well-known characteristic of autistic communication. Some autistic people say they avoid looking at faces because it is too difficult to process spoken language and confusing facial expressions at the same time. I think of eye contact as "conversational gaze" and prioritize it for certain situations.

If I am playing with a toy or doing a teaching activity with a child, I am content to have both of us focusing on the toy or task. However, if a child is making a request, directing an action or asking a question, I encourage looking, at least briefly, at the person who is expected to respond.

That "encouragement" would be different for each of the boys in this section. With Lucas, I would pause before responding and perhaps move a requested item closer to my face to get him to glance up and see why there was a delay. Seth can't see me, but he should learn to turn toward his listener when he speaks (instead of spinning around in circles), so I might gently touch his shoulder and turn him toward me. I would explain to Terek that when he is asking for something (object, action or information) or thanking someone, other people will respond faster and more willingly if he also looks at them.

Both natural conversation and eye gaze can be difficult to elicit from children on the autism spectrum, but it often goes better if you are easy to look at. If your facial expression is reliably calm, relaxed and slightly smiling, conversational gaze will be easier for the child.

Intonation

The speech of autistic people is sometimes described as robotic, monotone or mechanical. Improving prosody could be a long-term speech therapy project, but for frequently expected language such as the Pledge of Allegiance or "Good morning, Mrs. Anderson," try giving an exact model to imitate. This can also help when coaching the child for lines in a play or brief presentation. Tell the child "Say it like this," and demonstrate the appropriate intonation pattern. This will be much more effective than asking him to say it with feeling or with emphasis on certain words. Children with echoic tendencies may be especially adept at copying your intonation model.

Key points about teaching methods

One-to-one teaching

Young children with echolalia may need help learning to cooperate with direct instruction and guided play, much like children at the pre-symbolic level of communication. Ideas provided for Darius in Chapter 3 should be helpful here too. These children will be confused by multiple speakers in group discussions and are often distracted or anxious during group lessons. For new learning, many will benefit from one-to-one instruction followed by practice in more natural settings.

Visual schedules

Many autistic children are drawn to print, are very attentive to letters and numbers and even show the spontaneous reading of hyperlexia. Despite poor comprehension of stories, they will usually understand the concrete, predictable language of visual schedules using pictures, printed words or braille. Often, pictures are not needed on schedules for this group of children.

In a confusing world, a schedule is very helpful, not only for routines but to show changes in a concrete way. The child who constantly asks about a change to the schedule can learn to "Check the schedule" instead of asking the same question repeatedly. The teacher might need to offer an explanation once, add a brief note to the child's schedule such as "No field trip today because it is raining," and direct the child, verbally and with a gesture, to "Check the schedule." After saying this once or twice, a gesture toward the schedule should suffice. There is still some inconvenience involved, but it is better than having to stop and respond a dozen times to an anxious child who perseverates on saying "No field trip today? It's raining? No field trip?"

Children can also learn to follow some parts of the schedule independently, which is a valuable way to decrease prompt dependency.

Just start

"Just start" means that instead of waiting until a child can show you he is ready to work, or saying "If you don't...then you can't..." or otherwise getting into a power struggle, you just start the activity yourself. Frequently, the autistic child is resisting because he doesn't understand what is expected or doesn't believe he can do it.

Calmly and gently, just spin the spinner and move the game pieces, or do the first few math problems, or read the directions and answer the first question on the social studies paper. Then build in pauses and let the student finish an answer or move a game piece that you pretend you can't reach. Gradually let him take over and offer help when he is struggling.

Say "I'll help" to really mean you will give reassuring assistance. When children hear the words "I'll help," they should be thinking "Oh good, then maybe I can do it," not "Uh-oh, someone is going to force me to do it."

Reinforcement

Reward behaviors you want to see again but be cautious with praise. Try to give verbal approval in ways that will sound right if echoed. For example, if a child completes a puzzle and says "Yay, it's done!" because that is what you said yesterday, this is more accurate and appropriate than if he echoes your "Yay, you did it!"

We can reinforce children for not doing things as well as for doing things, but the expectations must be understood and must be something the child can do. Social narratives often explain incentive-based plans.

As described in Chapter 4, it is still important to "keep calm and carry on," use errorless learning, not confuse testing with teaching and not assume comprehension. In fact, do assume that comprehension is part of the problem, especially when dealing with echolalia and hyperlexia.

Language modeling

Modeling is especially good for echolalic children because of their strong tendency to imitate what they hear. But it's important to model language that is still appropriate when echoed and helps develop meaning for the child. The basics of language modeling are in Chapter 4. An expansion on modeling, especially for children who echo, is next.

Some of the suggestions I give most frequently to teams working with children who echo are:

- Don't ask so many questions, especially if the child doesn't answer questions yet. The child who echoes will soon sound as if everything he says is a question.

- Model language that will still be true and appropriate if echoed. "Time for the bathroom" works if he spontaneously says it to you later. But "Do you need to use the bathroom?" is confusing if the child later says it when trying to request a bathroom break.

- Model one- to three-word phrases at first, even if the child is echoing full sentences, and match them to what the child is experiencing. He needs the simplicity to connect the meaning with the words even though his memory allows him to repeat longer sentences.

- Use names instead of pronouns for a while to minimize the "I-you" confusion.

- Expect comprehension difficulties even if he can follow some directions. Children who understand language well do not echo, although young children typically do imitate key words a lot as they are learning to talk.

- Don't be afraid to model and practice the same things a lot. The more difficult skills may take a lot of repetition and autistic children are more comfortable with predictability than novelty.

- But watch out for associative patterns. If he says "Tie shoe" and you respond "Okay" a few times, he may start saying "Tie shoe okay." You may need to vary your response or just tie the shoe and say nothing to avoid confusing him.

For greetings, avoid prompting him to reply unless you are the one who greeted him. There shouldn't be a third person involved or he'll simply learn to wait for the outside prompter. If saying "Hi, Eric" gets no response or causes him to repeat "Hi, Eric" to you, get his attention before the greeting. Say "Eric!" and when he looks up, then say "Hi!" He will probably say "Hi" back to you, without including his own name. Often, you will also get good eye contact.

Teach this technique to other people who greet him often. If he does not respond, prompt the other person to say "Eric!" and then when he alerts, say "Hi," "Hello," "Good morning" or "Bye." He will probably echo the greeting he hears, without attaching his own name. If he does not respond, simply say the greeting word again, in a friendly but assertive tone. This tends to work faster with "Bye" than with "Hello," possibly because "Goodbye" signals a more precise event—someone is leaving.

To get him to add the other person's name, practice in a group where one person greets several children before him, and he hears each one say "Hi, Mrs. Smith" after she says "Hi" and each child's name. However, the first focus should be that he responds without echoing his own name.

Some things get better without direct instruction. If articulation is poor and the child's speech is unclear, it often improves greatly as more conventional language is acquired and the child understands what he is saying.

Delayed echoing of books and movie scripts also decreases as more conventional language develops, or it can be addressed more directly later with an incentive plan, as described for Seth in Chapter 6.

Say "Let's..." or "Time to..." instead of "Can you...?" when possible ("Let's sing a song"; "Time to close the door...take a bath," etc.) as it will be more appropriate when he re-uses it. It is also a bit less apt to elicit the "automatic No!"

Saying "No thank you!" when you mean "Don't do that!" is not, in my opinion, a more polite way to prohibit a behavior. And it certainly is not seen as polite when children copy the pattern and say "No thank you!" to an adult's directions.

Avoid language that is not exactly what you mean or not true. "I'll help" should mean he will benefit from your assistance, not that you will take something he doesn't want to part with or make him do something or go somewhere. It would be better to just say "...or I'll take it" if that is what you mean.

Behavior

The issues described in the behavior section of Chapter 4 are still relevant. After all, the children in this group still have autism.

Like others on the autism spectrum who are at earlier or later stages of development, they may show distress at transitions, new activities or changes of routine; development of time-consuming rituals; resistance to adult direction; eating and sleeping disorders; perseverative actions such as flipping, flapping, flushing, spinning, switching and slamming. Their play is often solitary, stereotypical, perseverative and repetitive. They may engage adults in excessive, repetitive verbal interactions and almost always prefer interacting with adults rather than children.

But now that they are talking, some other behaviors may

become more obvious, such as the "automatic No!" response, verbal perseveration and echoes that embarrass you.

The "automatic No!" generally starts as a defense against something the child finds alarming, but it can grow into a strong resistance to even mild expectations. Verbal/vocal perseveration has always seemed to me to be a similarly automatic, unplanned behavior that the child may not even be aware he is doing. I believe it functions to drown out confusion, provide distraction and reduce anxiety; as if the child is thinking "That bothers me, and this comforts me, so I will do it." Sometimes it may just be an enjoyable form of self-entertainment.

Angry echoes may sound as if the bad behavior is coming from you. Consider the child who screams "Don't hit me!" as he is hitting you. Words and sounds that are R-rated may be echoed from bits overheard on television or from the parents' bedroom. Don't take any of this personally. When possible, laugh.

Tracking progress

Consider why you are doing this work. If it is for research, including in-treatment research to improve evidence-based practice, you will need data that is specific and precise and relevant to the study.

Even without the requirements of research, you need to be able to measure what you are teaching, determine if there has been progress, note any positive or negative side effects and explain what the results mean. As discussed in Chapter 4, different goals lend themselves to different types of measurement. Here are some sample ideas for the children in this group:

• Language sampling is a good way to measure the progress Lucas makes in using conventional communication. You can count the frequency and percentage of accuracy in his use of "I want," relevant comments, protests and directives. If done through video recording, you could also document the variety of toys he used and the varied ways he learned to play with them.

+ In a practice session for requesting during a snack, use a checklist of times he used "I want" in imitation or spontaneously, and the times he used an echoic form such as "You want a cracker?" Spontaneous requests would be those in which he said "I want (name of a snack)" without immediately imitating exactly what another person had just requested. Measure progress as a percentage of spontaneous requests as compared with his total number of attempts.

+ A chart of accuracy would be an easy way to track Seth's progress on answering yes/no questions. With a column for answers that should be "yes" and one for those that should be "no," you can simply use a plus or minus sign to indicate his accuracy. If you do ten or 20 questions, it will be easy to obtain a percentage.

+ For Terek's upsets at school, keep a running record for a week or a month and track the percentage that resulted in outbursts or that he handled with prompted or spontaneous appropriate language.

+ In a report to parents or a team, any data should be accompanied by a narrative that describes the meaning of the results and other relevant information such as: "Although he likes all three choices, Lucas gets stuck on asking for the same snack repeatedly" or "Terek manages outbursts better in the morning; he still needs prompts 40% of the time to clearly state his problem."

Generalization

Typically, skills learned in a natural context, as supported by most of the goals for Lucas and for Seth's travel routes, will generalize to spontaneous use most readily because there is little difference between the teaching situation and the real-life use. Lessons learned sitting at a table may require deliberate practice in natural settings. Some skills grow on their own, such as using yes/no with questions other than those practiced. Practiced and reinforced behaviors, such as Seth's inhibition of chanting or Terek's self-control when upset, will often need to be given boosters of reinforcement in other settings.

Most students I've known, from pre-symbolic to highly verbal, have enjoyed doing the independent work described in Chapter 6, and it has generalized well to other settings, as long as the familiar set-up and process are maintained. Even non-speaking, easily agitated children have been able complete a sequence of independent tasks in mainstream classrooms or other busy places.

What if they are already adults?

We hope that echolalia will be resolved long before adulthood, but if not, modeling and instruction of the basic functions of communication can still be useful. Language modeling can be incorporated into daily living and recreational activities for people of any age, initially using single words and short phrases that are age-appropriate.

Certainly, there are adults with language abilities who have not progressed beyond the level Terek is using in Chapter 6, but they too can extend and broaden their communication abilities to enhance the quality of their adult lifestyles. Finding ways to increase independent activity and social interaction continue to be valuable and appreciated.

Progress may be slower for adults, but learning is a lifelong activity.

Bottom line

Progress in communication for autistic children needs work even if they are speaking clearly. Language is vital to literacy, education and interaction. Echolalia is an especially divergent language acquisition path not often seen outside of autism. Children may, or may not, find their own way out of echolalia, but don't wait and see. Time lost is not coming back.

PART III

ADVANCED LANGUAGE WITH GAPS

Chapter 8

Early Gaps

Mia

Speaking clearly, with excellent grammar and syntax and an impressive vocabulary should mean no communication problems, right? But even the autistic students who have the most advanced speech and language abilities have difficulties with communication that negatively impact their lives. The gap between their intellectual knowledge and their personal interactions can be especially startling when they present as highly intelligent but speak in ways that seem rude or misunderstand figurative language and monopolize conversations with monologues on obscure topics. The "gaps" in their advanced language can outweigh their intellectual strengths as they try to move through life comfortably.

As compared with less capable students on the autism spectrum, they are more likely to be blamed for their social deficiencies. Surely if she knows all the constellations in the sky, she must know better than to abruptly walk away when a new person is introduced to her, right?

We, of course, know that social interaction is a major deficit area of the autism spectrum. We have seen it in the diagnostic criteria and in the play and interaction of the six children in the preceding chapters. Many books and articles have been written about the problem and ways to teach appropriate social skills. Therapists, parents and teachers pour hours of dedicated effort into helping autistic children and adults to improve their social interaction behaviors. No doubt, the children or adults you know have been exposed to individual or group intervention for social skills. It is a big job, a long job, an important job. And social interaction has a tremendous impact on the ability of people on the autism spectrum to acquire and keep friends and employment.

This book is not a course in social skills or social understanding, but this section will address some of the common communication-based behaviors that adversely affect social interactions.

First, some common characteristics. Many highly verbal people on the autism spectrum:

+ are more interested in facts than in the opinions of others, are highly invested in being "right" and are not inclined toward compromise

+ appear egocentric, which is not surprising because both "ego" and "aut" mean self. They are not neurologically "wired" for easy, natural perspective taking and empathy, although some have a strong desire to make the world a better place. Honesty and tenacity are common traits

+ speak with intonation and word choice that others consider rude. Sometimes these are exact repetitions or modifications of scoldings, protests or arguments they have heard from annoyed adults

+ cannot readily interpret the meaning of facial expressions, shared glances, eye rolls, tone of voice and gestures. Their own conversational gaze, intonation patterns, facial expression and body movements may be limited, stiff and unnatural

+ respond as if assaulted by sensory input from lights, sounds, smells and textures and may complain vigorously about this discomfort

+ misunderstand idioms, sarcasm, jokes and other non-literal language. Despite learning the meanings of specific idioms such as "under the weather" and "eats like a horse" in third grade and studying books of idioms with fascination, young adults may still struggle with newscasters and politicians who speak of "rattling sabers in a negotiation," "out there going rogue" and "whether this is just a one-off"

• prefer reading nonfiction (facts) rather than fiction (feelings, relationships, deliberate deception) and have better comprehension of nonfiction

• are not easily able to make or keep friends

• are anxious, especially in social situations where much is uncertain and confusing, and are prone to explosive outbursts when overwhelmed. This is a sensitivity of most autistic people, and those with more advanced abilities are additionally challenged by being expected to function more independently in a wider, more complex and confusing range of society

• may avoid group activities and team projects, and rarely participate happily in team sports. Group activities can be noisy and confusing, team projects require compromise and shared roles, and team sports benefit from good motor coordination and ability to see the perspective of others. These are not ASD-friendly characteristics

• struggle with the "executive functions" such as planning and goal setting, organizing belongings and ideas, inhibiting impulses, initiating tasks, following through to completion, and managing time.

As adults, many of these communicative, social and cognitive characteristics adversely affect a person's ability to gain and retain employment. Consequently, many bright or brilliant autistic individuals remain unemployed or significantly under-employed. Surely this makes a dent in their safety, happiness, independence and productivity.

Although we cannot eliminate all the effects of autism, we can help children grow to manage and modify some of the characteristics that really impede their ability to sail their own ships.

In this chapter and the next one, Mia, Grady and Evan will tackle some of these tendencies and avoidances.

Mia

Mia is seven years old and attends second grade with 22 other children. Last year she had support from a paraprofessional during most first-grade activities. She had a successful school year, so her team decided she did not need continued one-to-one support. Her second-grade teacher has a classroom assistant whose attention is divided among Mia and three other children with learning differences.

Mia is academically ahead of her classmates in some things and behind in others. She reads and spells very well, and has great interest in unicorns, mermaids and vacuum cleaners. Not surprisingly, some of her favored reading materials are more available in second grade than others, so she brings her manuals and advertising brochures about vacuum cleaners to school. Mia plans to dress as a vacuum cleaner for Halloween.

With less adult support, Mia is struggling more this year. When listening to a chapter book and discussing the content in a large group, she is often fidgety and squirmy. Almost daily, Mia asks to go to the bathroom during read aloud or math instructions. Then she hasn't heard the story conversation or the math instructions and needs individual help from the teacher or assistant to do the related schoolwork.

This departure works well for Mia because she has trouble following the multiple steps of instructions the teacher gives to the class, is further confused by her classmates' questions, and benefits from the individual help given when she returns. But it is frustrating and time-consuming for her teachers. Some adults understand that Mia leaves at those times because she is confused by the instructions and needs to lower her anxiety. Others believe she does not understand the directions because she wasn't there to hear them.

Some other differences that complicate second grade for Mia (and consequently for her teachers and classmates) include:

- Mia desperately wants to be first in line, all the time, and creates minor chaos when she is not.

- She becomes very distressed if she loses a game or her answer is incorrect, occasionally flipping a game off a table or dashing out of the room.

- She covers her ears during unison recitations or singing, in which the children's voices are often not really all together, and she is upset by sudden or loud noises. Fire drills were especially alarming to her in kindergarten and she refused to come to school for a while to avoid them. After being promised that she would be warned in advance and taken outdoors before the alarm sounded, she became calmer and she is now able to tolerate the regular fire drill procedure.

- She is very invested in schedules and asks repeatedly about changes. During a spelling lesson she may remind the teacher that it is 11:15 and time for science.

- She has adequate math computation skills, and a fairly strong conceptual understanding of mathematics, but she struggles with word problems.

- She becomes very anxious if confused or uncertain of how to do something, and this can sometimes escalate to screaming or throwing papers and books.

- She is calmer and more productive during individual or self-guided instruction, such as on a computer, than in large group lessons or discussions. Mia has learned to do independent folder work, as described for Terek in Chapter 6. Working alone with these extended practice lessons is one of the most reliably calm periods of her school day. During independent work she knows what to do and she knows how to do it.

- She sings or hums to herself during whole class lessons.

- She wanders unproductively around the classroom during arrival and departure times even though the teacher has repeatedly gone over the expectations and most of the class now completes the routines independently. Mia cooperates when prompted by the teacher, but she still needs several verbal reminders to accomplish these daily expectations.

- She does not play or converse much with her classmates but has one "target friend," a girl named Yumiko who has very long shiny black hair, which Mia loves to touch. In addition to being a sensory attraction, Yumiko's distinctive hair helps Mia to identify her in a jumble of children. Yumiko, whose Japanese name means beautiful and helpful, is willing to patiently help Mia when she is confused by classroom expectations. Mia wants to be near Yumiko anytime the children are away from their desks.

- Mia is confused by non-literal language. When a classmate accused her of cutting in line, she replied indignantly, "I'm not cutting! I don't even have scissors!"

- She has learned not to blurt out answers without raising her hand, but often just raises her hand as she is blurting out an answer. She hasn't mastered the "wait to be called on" part.

Mia's new goals will address increasing her independence with the arrival and departure routines, helping her leave stressful situations more gracefully, developing her tolerance of losing and increasing her connection to her classmates. Several other issues will be addressed too.

Goal #1: Mia will follow the daily classroom procedures for arriving at, and leaving, school without reminders from her teachers.

For the morning routine, provide a list of the specific steps she needs to accomplish. If there are too many at present, just write down a few for now. For example, the list might be:

1. coat, hat and mittens in cubby

2. boots on floor of cubby

3. folder to Mrs. Putnam

4. backpack to Mrs. Salinas.

...and then Mrs. Salinas helps her unload the other items from her backpack and put them where they belong.

I'd suggest laminating the list to her desk. Let her check off completed items with a marker that can just be rubbed away for the next day.

Do a similar list for the afternoon departure routine. Although Mia can easily read them herself, read the lists together during the day and remind her that she can do these things independently so you will try not to talk to her while she does them. The absence of verbal prompts should be a familiar concept from her independent folder work. She may even remind you not to talk.

Concentrate on backing out of the prompting procedure immediately. The list is a valuable tool, and it needs to be seen as a script for her to memorize and follow. Therefore, the adult assistance should be as nonverbal as possible and should *not* include questions like "What should you do next?" Mia may wait for the adult to ask these questions, which practically precludes eventual independence. If she begins to wander, simply direct her to the list by pointing to it and saying something like "Number 3 is…" and let her fill in the expected action. Later, say nothing and just point to the paper. She should begin to follow the printed list herself and eventually just do the memorized routine independently.

It will be more motivating if you can have something at the end of the list that is both rewarding and productive for Mia. This might be "follow the directions to color the picture that's on your desk" in the morning or "look at your vacuum cleaner brochures" while waiting for the bus in the afternoon.

This goal is not about speaking or listening, but it is communication. Mia is developing early executive functions of organization and follow-through by way of written receptive language.

Goal #2: Mia will play three different games with one or two classmates at a time and will respond to winning or losing without behavioral outbursts.

An extreme need to win can be a challenging issue for students on the autism spectrum but avoiding the word "loser" and giving examples of a specific role for those who are not the winner often helps.

Write a brief social narrative about winning and being a good sport and things that each person could say at the end of the game. Here is a sample:

Playing games

When people play a game together, only one person wins. That person might say "I won!"

The people who did not win have a job at the end of the game. Their job is to be "good sports." The good sports can say things like "Congratulations!" or "It was a good game" or "Maybe I will win next time."

Another possibility is to teach her to just say "good game" and give a high five at the end of a game, regardless of who wins. This is simpler and can also be introduced with a social narrative:

Lots of children like to play games. Everyone likes to win but nobody wins every time. When the game ends, only the child who finished first says "I won!" But everyone who played the game can give high fives and say "Good game!"

Mia might listen attentively as you read it to her and even smile and say that she thinks it is a good idea. That does not, of course, mean that she will readily give up protesting when she loses, but it's a start. It is especially important that she has something to say when she does not win.

Practice playing games with her yourself before expecting her to do this with another child. When you do start including another child, you might want to ask the playmate to say "Good game!" instead of "I won!" or "You won!"—at least initially. Gradually increase the number of players and let the invited children respond naturally. Ideally, Mia will learn not to overreact to their comments and may begin to use some of them herself.

Review the social narrative about games with her occasionally, especially just before you play a game. When she wins, point out that you are being the "good sport" and say one of the example statements or something similar. If you win, model the use of "Good game!" instead of saying "I won."

With either plan, accepting loss is probably going to be difficult for Mia, so you may need to add an incentive. This might be five minutes' free reading time after she has successfully been a "good sport" or ended a game with "Good game!" regardless of whether she won or not.

Goal #3: When needing to leave a group lesson or other classroom

activity, Mia will follow a planned process for asking to leave instead of bolting out of the room.

Leaving the classroom is an accommodation offered to Mia that is not available to the other children in her class. It might seem unfair, but given her explosive tendencies, letting her leave is a benefit to the rest of the class, and I have rarely seen young children complain because their autistic classmate has expectations different from their own. They seem to readily recognize that children have different needs. If not, teachers can easily explain this to them. A brief explanation that children are working on many different things in second grade may suffice. In a longer discussion of personal differences, classmates may announce their own diagnoses or those of their siblings or cousins.

Help Mia learn to leave an activity peacefully and eventually to recognize that she needs to leave. This will be a valuable life skill as she grows.

If she says "I need to leave. It's too noisy," remember that this is much better than having a meltdown or bolting. Go with her to another activity or to another space to continue the same work. Ideally, this can happen within the classroom now that Mia does not have one-to-one support.

To help her learn to request a break, write the words "I need to leave" on a small card, show it to Mia and tell her she can say this anytime she feels the need for a break. Then, when a teacher observes that it would probably be a good time for her to leave, the teacher can simply slide the card in front of her and tap it. If she reads it, take her for the break; if she pushes it away or says "No thanks," accept it and move on unless you feel she really needs to go, in which case you can overrule her. After the process is familiar to Mia, tape the small card to her desk and just tap it as a suggestion when needed.

If she does stay and you know she is stressed, provide more help. She may use the card without prompting if it is just nearby and she knows how it works. The purpose is to provide her with an unspoken cue as a bridge to learning to make the spontaneous request. If you simply ask her if she wants to go, she may think she always needs to wait until it is suggested, and we want her to know she can advocate for this accommodation herself.

Have her attend large group lessons for those things she can do well and for other times that you think might be successful, but retreat early if necessary, so she doesn't practice inappropriate behavior. Do individualized pull-out instruction or independent work at times that she is chronically disengaged in the group.

React very little to her outbursts and sobs when you know what the problem is and that it will pass quickly. Sometimes she just needs a little space to get used to the idea that, for example, her partner is not Yumiko this time. This is often a good time to say "I will help" and just start the activity.

Goal #4: Mia will increase her interaction with her classmates by:

(a) interviewing classmates and, later, initiating conversations based on the information she knows about them and

(b) imitating adult models to issue invitations or make apologies.

Create a short written interview and practice it a few times with Mia. Then borrow one classmate at a time for her to interview in a corner of the room or out in the hall. I have not yet met a teacher who was unwilling to let students participate in this project. She can ask each child three or four questions that are not too personal but that provide information she can later use in conversation with them. Examples:

+ Do you have any pets?
+ What do you like to play at home?
+ What do you like to do at recess?
+ What is your favorite school lunch?
+ What do you like to read about?

End with "Do you want to ask me any questions?"

Maintain a relaxed, unhurried atmosphere, but don't expect these interactions to last long. Some of the interviews will go by very quickly and the other children may not ask questions, but some will at least ask her the same questions that she asked them, and a few will launch into stories about their pets or interests. Mia may spontaneously share information, perhaps telling everyone the same story about finding her goldfish belly up in the fishbowl. Although you may tire of hearing it, remember it is new to each of her classmates and gives her a comfortable topic to initiate.

The adult helper should keep a low profile and encourage Mia to track which students she has seen. Mia should invite the next one to come chat with her if the classroom teacher has not put restrictions on which children are available that day. It is important for the adult to keep notes about the children's answers. Sometimes the autistic child creates a notebook with pictures of each classmate and the child's responses to her questions. Other information can be added to a child's page as Mia learns it—for example, that Abram's dog had puppies or Carla's grandfather is moving in with her family. The interview information can also be graphed for a class presentation in which Mia demonstrates that French toast is the favorite school lunch or more children like the swings than the monkey bars or 14 of the 23 second-graders have a pet.

Graphing the data and presenting to the class can be a good learning experience, but it is more important to help Mia use the information to have casual conversations with her peers. Coach her to ask Abram how many puppies Zena had or tell Fiona that she got a new goldfish. Encourage her to congratulate Aadya for getting all the way across the monkey bars and to invite Jake to play the math game with her.

Sometimes just a nudge and a suggestion will be enough to help Mia initiate a conversation with another child, but sometimes she will need more direct and specific help. If she doesn't know how to congratulate Aadya, tell her exactly what to say and show her how to say it: "Hey, Aadya, you did all seven bars! That's great!" Be sure to model the intonation as well as the words. It will be much easier for

Mia to copy what she hears you say than to follow instructions to "Say it like you mean it."

Modeling the exact words and tone of voice can be especially helpful when coaching Mia through a conflict. She sometimes offends her classmates unintentionally by bumping into them as she rushes to be first in line, laughing when someone falls down or giggling when a classmate reads a sad journal entry. Tell her that even if it was an accident she should apologize, and then demonstrate how to do so. This may need to include going to the offended child instead of just echoing your apology model from afar. Examples:

- Go to Jeremy and say "I'm sorry I bumped you. I'll try not to go so fast."

- Tell Micah "I'm sorry you're sad. I didn't mean to laugh."

Modeling the exact words and tone of voice needed can also be effective when helping an autistic child deliver lines in a play convincingly or read aloud with appropriate intonation.

Other thoughts for Mia

Mia would benefit from inclusion in a social skills group to learn and practice better interactions with her peers. Some of her four suggested goals might be addressed though such a group.

She should also work on accepting that she cannot always be first in line or called on every time she raises her hand and that she should not hum or sing during class lessons. Of course, these were problems in kindergarten and first grade too, but Mia's paraprofessional helper managed them with prompts, assists and sometimes departure from the class. Now, she does not have such close supervision, and the behaviors seem even more inappropriate because she is older. Visual cues and reinforcement plans similar to those used in her Goal #3, Seth's Goal #1 and Terek's Goal #1 will be useful here.

Mia will need extra support with understanding figurative language and interpreting math word problems, and her reading comprehension should be closely monitored even though she is advanced in decoding. She will probably start studying idioms in third grade, but it is never too soon to start noticing and helping when she seems confused.

She should be encouraged to read and follow directions more independently, at least for familiar tasks, to skip questions she can't answer, to ask for help when needed and to wait patiently for a response.

As she progresses through the next few grades, Mia may continue to need lists and social narratives in new situations, additional help with graceful departures when she is stressed, and considerable support with peer interactions. In middle and high school, she may face some of the difficulties that Grady and Evan will address in Chapter 9.

Chapter 9

Still Some Gaps

Grady and Evan

Grady and Evan have strong speech and language skills with impressive vocabularies and extensive knowledge of many subjects. Grady has been especially interested in baseball statistics, planets and violent weather, while Evan gravitates toward art history and politics. Both have studied their favorite subjects in depth and are eager to talk about them, without much concern for their listeners' interest. Diagnostically, these are examples of the extreme interests associated with autism, which some people now refer to as "enthusiasms" (Prizant 2015, p.54).

Both boys attend regular education classes, with sporadic paraprofessional support. Although they have solid academic ability and above-average intelligence, they have gaps in social communication that significantly impact their school lives.

Grady

Grady attempts to do what's expected at school but can't always keep up with the level of independence, creative thought and flexibility required in middle school. He is tense and anxious much of the time in seventh grade. He no longer bolts out of the classroom when distressed, but he complains of illness often and asks to go home after minor upsets.

Sometimes he shouts or cries when more stressed. One time it went like this:

> Grady needed help with his essay, so he raised his hand and repeatedly called his teacher's name. She was helping another student and asked him to wait, but Grady continued to call to her. Exasperated, she said, "I'll get to you in a minute, Grady. I'm helping Tim. The world doesn't revolve around you, you know!" In a heartbeat, Grady replied, "I know. It doesn't revolve around you either. It revolves around the sun." For this, he earned a demerit, so he cried, screamed, "That's not fair!" and threw his books on the floor. In Grady's literal mind, he had just been stating an interesting fact in a conversation with his teacher. He had no idea that he was being disrespectful.

In earlier grades, Grady has worked on goals similar to Mia's with good results but lingering shadows. He can lose a game or wait to be called on in class, and no longer needs to be the first person out the door when the bell rings. But he may grumble quietly when his side loses a vote, or if he doesn't get selected to answer every time he raises his hand. When he gets a chance to talk in class, he may go on and on about a tangentially related topic.

Grady now quickly learns each year's new expectations around school arrival and departure, but like Mia he needed lists for several years in elementary school. He follows the complicated rotating class schedule independently, but the particulars of organization, such as arriving in a class with the appropriate books and materials, turning in homework and saving or discarding completed work as expected are still significant challenges for Grady.

He has difficulty working with small groups of classmates. Grady complains that they don't do their share and they often say the same of him. He has strong opinions and is not prone to compromising. He tells his teachers, "I would prefer to be a group of one."

He loves sharing his knowledge with his class, especially if it relates even tangentially to one of his "enthusiasms." So if the city of Atlanta is mentioned as the setting of a novel, for example, Grady may want to tell the class the history and statistics of the Atlanta Braves, including which years they played in which stadiums, who holds their home run record and when they won division titles.

Grady's goals focus on working in small groups with classmates, minimizing lengthy monologues during class discussions, expressing his distress more calmly and completing homework.

Goal #1: Grady will work productively with one to three classmates for science labs and small group projects.

Grady's teachers have tried to match him with partners and group mates who are strong students, have patient and helpful personalities, and recognize that Grady might need extra help. Nevertheless, problems often arise because Grady feels he needs to be in charge whether or not he fully understands the purpose or instructions of the project. Other times, he is uninterested in the task or offended by the grouping and wants to neither lead nor follow. Consequently, he may either lead the group astray and ignore their attempts to redirect him or avoid the exercise altogether and try to read from a personal book or unrelated computer sites.

Occasionally, the students in the group will find a solution themselves, but more often teacher intervention and close monitoring will be needed. Here are some things that help.

As an introductory overview, create a social narrative about the general basics of working with others, such as:

Working together

At school and in life we all do some things alone and some things with other people. Learning to work with others is an important part of a good education. Most adults need to work with others at their jobs. In seventh grade, students work with a lab partner in science and with two or three classmates for some school projects. When working with others it is important to:

- Be sure everyone understands what the whole group is trying to accomplish.

- Tell your ideas and listen to other students' ideas.

- Make a plan for who will do which parts of the work.

- Do your part of the work on time.

Review this with Grady several times in preparation for assigned group projects. Or use something similar with the whole class if appropriate. Continue to try to match him with students who will clearly understand the expectations and not be derailed if Grady is confused or overly directive. But don't overuse the same few group mates. Grady may also benefit from groupings of less academically inclined classmates if those groups are receiving more teacher assistance.

Assign specific roles to each student, or at least to Grady. It will be easier for him to let others participate if he knows that he is responsible for steps 1, 2 and 5 of the lab experiment, or that his job is to gather six facts about Chile's exports. Ideally, the group would organize a plan to share the workload, but for now Grady may be better able to accept the teacher's assignment than to make an agreement with his peers.

Check in frequently to see how the group is progressing and smooth any conflicts. Reinforce Grady's progress verbally or perhaps with a checklist that leads to a reward when he completes his tasks.

Goal #2: During classroom discussions, Grady will self-limit his monologues or respond to a pre-planned cue to end one.

Grady's tendency to monologue is at its worst when he is talking about one of his favorite interests, but he can also hijack the class discussion by providing an excess of factual information about a wide variety of topics. He is not trying to disrupt the lesson or keep the teacher from getting to the points she feels are important. Grady reads extensively on a variety of nonfiction topics and is just eager to share what he knows with his teacher and peers. He may even believe that he is responsible for enhancing their education, in the same way that he feels duty-bound to correct his teachers when they accidentally misstate a fact, mispronounce a word or misplace a comma.

Nevertheless, the whole class cannot be expected to wait for Grady to expound on everything he knows about sea life while the planned lesson on whale hunting floats listlessly in the air. In several conversations with the teacher, Grady has agreed that he should not monopolize a class discussion, but his actual behavior has not changed. It is very difficult for Grady to know how much is too much, but he, like Terek in Chapter 6, has worked in speech/language therapy on staying on the topic. The goal here is to help him see a discussion as a conversation among a group of people and to learn not to monopolize it or digress from the main topic.

First, put it in writing. A social narrative, printed out and reviewed with Grady occasionally at home and before class, will be more effective than an oral conversation. Here is a sample:

Discussions in the classroom

During class discussions, the students in seventh grade are expected to listen when classmates are talking, share information about the topic being discussed and allow time for others to talk.

If someone is talking too long, others will not have a turn, so the teacher will do one of these things:

- Say "Thank you for your contribution" and invite another student to speak.

- Say "That's getting away from the topic. We are discussing..." and invite another student to speak.

- Say "It's time for someone else to have a turn" and invite another student to speak.

If the teacher invites another student to speak or if the teacher starts talking about the topic when you are talking, it is time to sit down and listen.

Extrinsic reinforcement may be needed for this and for all of Grady's goals, so developing a simple token economy could be helpful. A token economy is a system of reinforcement in which students are given an immediate symbol (token) of reward (such as a ticket, star or check mark) for specific desirable behaviors and can later exchange the accumulated tokens for a tangible reward.

For Grady, the token economy might include rewards for meeting all four of his goals. It might look like this:

Some things need to change

Sometimes things need to change so that school will go better for you and everyone else. Everyone at school is learning and sometimes it is hard work. Here is a plan for helping you with some of your learning goals:

You can earn points for some school accomplishments and then trade the points for (a reward from home, currency for the school store, coupons for free reading or computer time, etc.). These are the ways you can earn a point:

- Do one of your assigned tasks while working in a group or with a partner.

- Redo a paper to correct mistakes or write a new draft.

- Contribute to a class discussion and sit down quietly when the teacher indicates your turn to talk is finished. Earn a bonus point when you stop before the teacher says your turn is finished.

- Ask to go to a quiet space or use a "problem page" instead of asking to go home.

- Complete a homework assignment. Earn a bonus point if no one needed to remind you to do it.

Goal #3: Grady will communicate his distress and negotiate a solution instead of having an emotional outburst or asking to go home when he is upset but not ill.

Grady has a history of school refusal, starting as an attempt to avoid fire drills in elementary school. With gradually decreasing accommodations in kindergarten through grade two, he, like Mia, eventually learned to tolerate the regular routine of fire drills. He was also upset by coming to school late, such as after a doctor's appointment, because the class would be at a different point in the daily routine. Following some dismissals because of behavior in fourth grade, he began to ask to go home when he was distressed and soon found this to be more effective if he complained of a stomach ache or headache.

To help Grady begin to face, rather than flee from, school upsets, recognize when he is overwhelmed and provide him with a simpler, more predictable and less demanding environment. This might be a break in the nurse's office, an option to do his work in the library, a short walk with a paraprofessional or a retreat to a sensory room. He will respond better if these are suggested as ways to help him feel better. Grady tends to automatically resist if he is commanded to leave when he is starting to become disruptive. If Grady's outbursts were more frequent and severe, even creating a part-time "office" for him in a quiet part of the school could be considered.

Develop a simple narrative explanation and a predictable solution such as:

Staying at school

Sometimes things happen at school that upset me. I get upset when I lose something or when someone says things I don't like or when I don't understand the work.

When I am upset it sometimes makes me feel sick and I want to go home so I can feel better. Students go home when they are sick with something caused by germs. Students do not go home when they are upset by something that happened at school, but sometimes they need a grown-up to help them find a way to feel better at school.

I can ask a grown-up to help me when I am upset at school. I can use a "problem page" to help explain what made me upset and to find a way to make it better. My parents and teachers want me to be safe and calm and happy and productive all day at school. I want that too. We will try to work on it together.

Problem page

I am upset because:

1. I lost...

2. I don't have...

3. I need...

4. A person named _____ said...

5. A person named _____ did...

6. I said or did something I wish I did not say or do. That thing was...

7. I am worried or upset about...

Because of what happened, I think this will happen:

_____

I would like to talk to: _____

To feel better, I need to:

- Go read in the library.
- Take a short walk.
- Go work in...
- Give or hear an apology.
- Get help with...

Grady will need help using these problem pages for a while, but it is a good step toward thinking through an issue and responding logically instead of falling apart.

Goal #4: Grady will reliably complete modified homework assignments and revisions.

Grady readily shares a lot of reasons why he believes he should not do homework, including:

- He works hard at school, and school has no business following him home.

- The teacher would know how smart he is if she would just call on him every time he raises his hand.

- If he has shown he can do it once or twice, that should be enough.

- He has other priorities at home—that is, studying his enthusiasms or playing video games.

- He shouldn't have to write essays because he doesn't want to be an author.

- He certainly shouldn't have to do over work that was incorrect. In his mind, done is done.

In reality, Grady is smart in many ways, but there are gaps in his intellect. When he does do homework, after much protest and delay, his parents often have to explain the expectations and help him organize the work, especially with writing assignments. And Grady often believes that his parents don't really know what the teacher wants, leading to more battles.

Also, Grady needs to practice the life skills of doing things in one setting to make progress in another and correcting mistakes. Part of doing homework is learning to remember and act on something that must be done here and now so that you will be prepared there and later. Homework can be important preparation for life.

That said, some accommodation and support are needed for Grady to make progress on this goal.

Grady's parents have dealt with homework resistance for years and have established a routine time and place for him to work on it, but struggles continue. He does get some of his homework done in a supported study hall on three days of the week. Some possibilities for dealing with the rest of it include the following.

Since Grady is familiar with the independent folder work that was described in Terek's goals (Chapter 6), make some of the schoolwork he does at home into independent work. This would need to be self-limited papers and worksheets that you are sure he can do without help.

For tasks he has real difficulty completing (or starting) by himself, give assistance in the supported study or resource room instead of expecting him to work on it at home.

Where quantity is a problem, consider modifications such as only expecting him to do the odd-numbered problems or a "no homework pass" if he can demonstrate the skill to his teacher.

Use notes, email or telephone contact with his parents to clarify expectations and to monitor the degree of assistance he needs with assignments. The help Grady receives from his parents may mask some of his difficulties with comprehension, so it is important to know how much help he needed. Using information shared by his parents, his teachers will better understand which aspects of learning are more difficult for Grady. For example, his parents might report that he independently answered the first five social studies questions correctly, but needed considerable help with the sixth one: "Why did the native Americans keep moving west?" This could be because the factual answers to the earlier questions could be found by matching them to the text, but the sixth answer required extrapolating meaning that wasn't specifically stated in the book.

Another complication of the homework issue is that Grady does not write things in his assignment book and often forgets to take home the books he needs for homework. He also stuffs papers haphazardly into his backpack and locker, and doesn't know which completed papers to save and which he can discard. When he has done his homework, he often forgets to turn it in to the teacher. Grady's disorganization is epic, even compared with the typical disorder of middle school students' lives. Obviously, he will need a lot of assistance with organization, as well as other executive functions, but we will focus on the use of the assignment book, an important form of written communication from Grady to himself. A few quick tips:

• Put the dates on the pages ahead of time, perhaps for a week at a time. He might like to do this at home or on Monday morning. A red day-and-date stamp would be visually distinct and require no handwriting.

• Teach him to write something after every class, even if just a straight line to mean no homework, in that class's section of the page.

• Develop easy abbreviations such as "pp" for pages and "?s 1–30 odd" to mean "Do all the odd-numbered problems between numbers 1 and 30."

• Teach him to highlight the assignments that require him to take home a book (or provide a set of books for home).

• When a teacher or assistant checks at the end of the day, reward Grady through his token economy for using his assignment book.

• While helping him, don't ask questions; just use a simple script that sounds as if he's talking to himself such as "Social studies is ending...gotta write down the assignment...gonna need the book...better highlight it." Avoid questions so he won't wait passively for them; with the script, you can drop out parts and let him fill them in to remind himself.

• Offer reinforcement as a part of his token economy program.

Grady could earn points for completing homework, for remembering to turn it in on time, or for doing the assignment independently.

Other thoughts about Grady

Grady sometimes says "Okay" or answers "Yes" when asked if he understands, without actually understanding. It is important to monitor his level of comprehension and independence with his academics. There will be times when he understands a concept and procedure well enough that he could teach it to the class, but other times he may miss important steps or not fully grasp the underlying concept. It is important for his teachers and parents to monitor which lessons he is understanding well enough that he can use them independently and generalize them to similar situations.

If you have to repeatedly keep telling him the same information, such as the steps for a math procedure, write it out for him and just point to the next step on the list instead of telling him orally each time. Then just let him follow the written steps and he will soon memorize them.

Grady loves to tell jokes but does not always understand why they are funny. Teach him a repertoire of appropriate jokes, demonstrating the timing and intonation, and explaining why they are funny. Study comic strips together and discuss what makes them humorous. As with idioms, Grady may still not always "get" new ones, but he can learn to ask a trusted adult or peer to explain figurative language.

It is inherent in Grady's diagnosis that he has legitimate difficulty understanding the needs and feelings of others. Consequently, I would deal directly with immediate interpersonal problems by telling him what to do as a practical solution ("Ask John to put his books on the other side of him") rather than questioning feelings ("How would you feel if John yelled at you because your books were in his way?") in confrontational situations. He does have a real need for help in understanding the feelings of others, but this can be better worked on in neutral practice situations with stories, videos, role playing and discussion. You could also tell him how others are feeling as he observes real-life events, but for now I'd avoid expecting him to figure out, or even accept, other people's emotions in the midst of his own stressful situations.

And, of course, Grady needs work on many other aspects of social interaction with peers and adults and on life skills such as helping with meal preparation, laundry and yard work, and navigating around his community.

Evan

Evan is a 15-year-old tenth-grader who was not diagnosed with autism until sixth grade. He likes to go to school but not to do homework, and he laments a lack of friends but may turn away social opportunities and avoid situations where he might feel awkward. After seeing a movie with others, he might say, "Sometimes I don't understand; I just laugh when they do."

In school he excels academically, despite some continued resistance to homework that does not interest him and a tendency to procrastinate on writing assignments and then get bogged down trying to find just the right words. He does not attempt to take notes in class or when reading, but generally gets by on his exceptional memory for information he reads or hears. His parents still do a lot of structuring, assisting and bribing to get him to complete assignments, but he will spend hours researching and studying a topic that interests him.

He has maintained an email relationship with a friend who moved away and has been to at least one school dance and danced with a girl. But other teens are generally a challenge for Evan as he does not reliably recognize and interpret the fast-paced slang, humor, sarcasm or flirtatiousness of his contemporaries. Evan understands the difference between literal and figurative language, and he has studied books of idioms and body language and has practiced picking out sarcasm in videos. He likes to use figurative language and can readily define similes and metaphors. He often uses familiar expressions accurately and has even created a few of his own. Evan once reported that some teasing students left him "steaming like a bag of vegetables in the microwave." But he still struggles with the many variations of these non-literal communication forms in daily life, and he often laments, "Why can't people just say what they mean?"

On one occasion last year he was the victim of a malicious prank. This was a case of outright bullying, and Evan was justifiably upset. But often Evan misinterprets the words and actions of his peers, thinking they are being friendly when they are teasing him or that they are harassing him when they are trying to be friendly. He might think a friendly peer who drapes an arm around his shoulders or gives him a congratulatory thump on the back is threatening him. He believes that the extraneous noises his classmates make by tapping pencils, scraping chairs and clearing their throats are deliberate attempts to annoy him. Sometimes he is correct.

Evan has a rather low opinion of other students' intelligence, especially if they disagree with him. He prefers interacting with adults, saying, "They know more than the kids do." Also, adults tend to be more appreciative of his favorite art and politics topics, and more willing to listen politely to his lengthy opinions. Adults are often impressed with Evan's obvious intelligence, but they are also the ones most likely to complain that he is rude.

He has made comments that were demeaning to other students, and retorts or demands that his teachers and other adults perceive as rude. This is very common among bright students on the autism spectrum, who often respond to frustration and anxiety by reverting to words and intonations that they remember hearing and associate with being upset. Often, these are exact repetitions of phrases and intonation that they have heard angry adults direct to them or their peers. Rudeness is a lesser evil than the screaming, slamming and physical aggression that accompany stress for many people on the autism spectrum, but it certainly interferes with social and workplace acceptability.

Evan has some ritual compulsions related to cleanliness such as not wanting others to touch his food, showering twice daily and washing his hands a lot. He is not especially interested in learning the life skills of adulthood like cooking, driving, managing finances or home and yard care. He is comfortable with letting his parents take care of him indefinitely and seems to see it as their job.

Evan's parents have tremendous understanding of his needs, abilities and limitations, and provide him with the structure, accommodation and monitored independence he needs to flourish developmentally. They learned long ago, for example, that if they didn't follow a precise series of steps for repairing discord, Evan would not be able to move on from the problem. They provide him with the "down-time," accepted foods, tag-less shirts, social support and other requirements that help minimize stress and keep him functioning fairly well. They recognize the incongruities in his reasoning and are justifiably concerned that he could easily be victimized. But they believe that he should be striving for more independence and are consciously planning ways to help him become a safe, happy, productive adult.

When comfortable, or excited about a topic, Evan can converse intelligently and enthusiastically. He has his favorite subjects, of course, but enjoys sharing information on a wide range of topics. However, he also has a history of selective mutism. In sixth grade, he stopped talking in several school settings which jump-started the evaluation that eventually led to his autism diagnosis. The selective mutism has resolved, but it is very difficult for Evan to converse freely about his hopes, anxieties, future plans or even likes and dislikes. When his parents or teachers attempt to discuss personal matters with him, Evan usually responds with "I don't know" or, if it sounds remotely like a reprimand, "I don't want to discuss it!"

Evan has no experience with volunteering or paid work outside his home. Although he will almost certainly go to college after high school, he has never spent a night away from his parents. Difficulties with goal setting and follow-through, social anxiety, inadequate interpretation of interpersonal interactions, low physical energy, sensory defensiveness and atypical diet and sleep patterns are likely to impact both his college experience and employment.

Some of Evan's communication issues that will be addressed in this chapter include decreasing rude comments and demands, increasing ability to explain his preferences and stressors, and developing ommunication skills needed for employment. A personal token economy system, not known to his classmates, provides Evan with some incentive for change.

> **Goal #1**: Evan will (a) accept being told that he has been rude and readily apologize, and (b) will imitate a modeled sample of "a better way to say it" half of the time.

Evan states that he doesn't always know he's being rude or can't control his rudeness. Accept that this is true but help increase his awareness. For now, work on rudeness through rewards for inhibiting it, helping him learn to stop and apologize, and teaching him ways to get his needs expressed without being rude. Even though he is an intelligent young man, it is very difficult for him and others on the autism spectrum to interpret what others consider rude, so it will be very helpful to tell him when he is rude and demonstrate other exact words and tones to use instead.

Address the rudeness issues, as privately as possible, by telling him that what he said was rude, unkind or inappropriate and why. Then give him an example of a way to say it better, modeling both the words and the intonation. He is more likely to accept this if you can also tell him why it will be better for him if he says it the way you modeled. For Evan, a particularly potent reason to avoid or apologize for rudeness is that people are more likely to do what he wants if he asks politely. If he immediately imitates your model, thank him and move on, but don't insist that he do so. This is easier in one-to-one situations, but rudeness is also likely to occur in a classroom, where you might need to address it immediately. Everyone probably already heard what he said anyway and will be watching to see how the teacher responds.

Create a social contract:

Repairing rudeness

Sometimes it is difficult to know what other people think is rude, but if someone tells you that you were rude, it nearly always helps to apologize. This is an important skill that will help you in school, with friends and in jobs.

In your token economy, you can earn a point for immediately saying something like "I'm sorry. I didn't mean to be rude" when a teacher says that something you said was rude or not okay at school.

You can earn a point for each class in which no rudeness concerns were noted.

You can earn an extra point if a teacher says "This would be a better way to say it," and gives you an example and you immediately repeat the words and tone of the example.

Since he will not easily generalize from one situation to another without a lot of practice, and not all teachers will want to participate, consider this a long-term project, not a quick fix.

Goal #2: Evan will share information about the strength of his likes and dislikes, preferences and stressors by responding to structured interviews.

Evan does not provide much information when asked what he likes about school or what stresses him during the day or what he wants people to know about him. This may not be because he is unwilling to share information; quite possibly, he hasn't sorted and connected the related bits of information or just can't add them up and organize a response. When he can't respond well to open-ended questions, try some "structured interviews."

Structured interviews can help you learn Evan's reactions to specific classes, behaviors of other students, difficult parts of his day, the strength of his ASD characteristics and how much importance he attaches to different expectations. Make a list of information you need or specific questions you want to ask before you begin. Maintain a calm, listening attitude during the interview without making judgments about his responses.

Start by saying you want to interview him and will be writing down the important things he tells you. Then try any of these samples that look promising:

- You could ask him to describe what a really good school day, or an especially bad one, would be for him. If this is still too open-ended, you may be able to help him along with starter sentences such as "First you wake up..." or "And then at the bus stop..." Sometimes describing a day provides organizational structure because he is following along a familiar time schedule, a list of events that are firmly in his memory. But the positives or negatives he mentions can tell you a lot about how he is processing his world. Does he perceive a really good day at the bus stop as one in which kids greet him and someone invites Evan to share a seat, or is it a day when everyone stands silently in line waiting for the bus and no one bothers him?

Or you could ask him specific questions about features of the day and let him respond on a scale as in these examples:

- On a scale of 1–5, how important are these to you:
  - Having time to work alone with a teacher.
  - Getting good grades.
  - Being able to move around often.

- Are these statements true, false, sort of true or very true about you:

  - You like to eat many different foods.

  - You like libraries, maps and computers better than ball games and rock concerts.

  - You are often awake or asleep at different times from the rest of your family.

- Are these things good or bad or okay? This can be done orally or with thumbs up, down or sideways for neutral.

  - Loudspeaker announcements.

  - Free reading time.

  - Class dismissal bells.

  - Hallways between classes.

  - Science class.

  - Group projects.

  - No-school days.

- Tell me three good things about school and three things you would like to change about school.

Whether you use one of these sample formats or a procedure such as "Which one of these is better/best?" or "Complete this sentence," practice with factual answers first to be sure Evan knows the type of response needed.

When you can have easy, open-ended discussions with Evan, there is no need for these techniques. But if not, 15 or 20 structured interview questions can often give you a clearer window to his thoughts, especially if he adds specifics when you ask "Can you tell me more about that?"

Sometimes an answer will seem odd to you and turn out to be a misunderstanding. For example, you might ask why he gave "knowing the schedule" an importance score of only 2 although he recites it daily and reminds you of it often. Evan's reply of "Because I already know the schedule" suggests he means he doesn't have to worry about it rather than that it is not important to him.

Goal #3: Evan will acquire four new communication/executive function skills specifically related to volunteer work and employment.

Evan will certainly go to college and perhaps graduate school, but he needs work skills too, and it is not wise to assume he will just understand employment expectations when his education is completed. From a communication point of view, work is another laboratory for developing interpersonal and executive function skills.

He may not be enthusiastic about a volunteer job. It would be wonderful if Evan was willing to volunteer for altruistic reasons, but if not, his parents might agree to pay him. Ideally, look for a position that fits with some of his interests and might set him up for paid part-time employment in a year or two or during college. He is not likely to want significant physical labor and can't tolerate cooking smells and busy, crowded places. Evan might like to usher at a community theater, help in a museum or library, walk dogs or follow a map and script to deliver campaign flyers.

If he volunteers at a library, his four mini-goals for work might be to:

+ greet or respond to patrons and know how to direct them to the restrooms and help desks

+ arrive on time, dressed appropriately, and come and go from breaks on time

+ use the break room to relax, read, chat a little with other workers and eat in the company of others

- develop and maintain a folder of his personal job responsibilities, including how to accomplish the expected behaviors and reminders such as not to say "excuse me" and then push aside patrons while he is shelving books. His folder should list the people he can go to if he has a problem, and samples of polite ways to initiate resolution. It could also include suggested topics to chat about in the break room.

Very little of this will just happen on its own. Unless the volunteer work is part of his school day, Evan's parents will need to help a lot with practicing these skills and developing the folder.

At the library, he will need a mentor to both show and tell him how to do his job. Explaining it in a meeting or just having him observe may not suffice. If it is not pointed out to him, he may see that the library worker put the books in alphabetical order, but not that she waited while someone finished looking at the books in that section. He should know that wherever he is in the library, he can respond with "The restrooms are on the first floor across from the elevator." He doesn't need to figure out the exact route to the restrooms from all parts of the library. He needs to know when to take his break, whether to ask permission or tell someone he is going and what time he should return to work.

Volunteer work, and later part-time employment will be very valuable steps toward launching him into adulthood.

Other thoughts about Evan

Note taking

Evan does not attempt to take written notes during lecture classes. Although he remembers a lot, he is not able to reliably recognize what is most important in a lecture. Evan says, "If the teacher said those things, he must think they are important." Handwriting is difficult for him and he feels he should write down every word, so he generally won't try to take notes.

Evan would benefit from some specific tutoring in note taking, perhaps from a resource-room teacher or speech/language pathologist. In the meantime, he could practice by:

+ having a copy of the teacher's notes to highlight during the lecture

+ getting a copy of a classmate's notes to review and highlight later

+ learning to just copy what the teacher writes on the board

+ typing on a computer instead of writing by hand, unless access to the computer causes him to stray off to other sites

+ highlighting key parts of passages in magazines and copies of text.

Some of these may be accommodations he can request in college. Of course, he will be able to highlight in his textbooks when he owns them, but Evan is firmly opposed to marring a book with notes, highlighting or underlining. It would be good to practice, perhaps starting with magazines.

Non-literal language

Figurative language and the meaning of gestures and facial expression are still difficult for Evan. Even when the words are literal, he may not grasp the underlying intent. He walked into a steakhouse that offers peanuts for customers while they are waiting for a table. Evan asked the cashier how much the bags of peanuts cost. She told him they were free, so he took two bags and went home.

He has had a lot of direct instruction in figurative language and nonverbal communication, and could benefit from more, especially as relates directly to teenagers' language and actions. But Evan may always need help translating non-literal information.

Emotional support at school

Although he generally maintains self-control at school, it is still an anxiety-provoking situation and he deserves some emotional assistance.

Try to view your role as supporting Evan in his attempts to cope and protecting him from becoming overwhelmed and having emotional meltdowns. Getting the work done is Evan's responsibility, whether he does it sooner or later. You do not need to push him to work at school, but a gentle nudge could help.

Recognize that it is sometimes difficult for him to start an in-class assignment. As he says, he needs time to gather his "thoughts and courage" to start something new. He may be unsure of what to do or simply unmotivated to do the task.

Since you may not always know which factors are involved, you can give him some time and see if he self-starts. Then offer to help him go over the directions or suggest a way he could start, but don't be offended if he says no. It will probably be counter-productive to coax or insist that he start the assigned work, but you may be able to give him a jump-start by providing him with an outline or graphic organizer. If all else fails and it is acceptable to the teacher, suggest that, for now, he could do some other schoolwork instead, or that he could go work in another space.

If you feel Evan should leave a class because he is getting upset, and he does not recognize this himself, say something supportive and say it calmly. Example: "This is a good time for a break in the guidance office."

Remember that crowded situations like assemblies and the cafeteria are difficult for Evan and he may choose to avoid them or need extra moral support and easy escape options.

Life and executive skills

If he is going to sail his own ship independently, Evan needs to acquire many more home and community life skills and improve his executive functioning skills. For college, he will especially need better ability to plan and initiate tasks, organize time and materials, and persist to reach goals.

Chapter 10

Advanced Language with Gaps: Expanded

The ability to speak clearly on factual topics is an asset we admire, and the world needs the knowledgeable contributions of people on the autism spectrum. But some of their communication characteristics attract negative attention. When they are confused by non-literal language, facial expressions and gestures or the meaning of jokes, autistic students appear naive. When they respond with rudeness, aggression or endless argument, they may be seen as annoying and selfish or even a bit scary.

School is a laboratory for learning about people and life, not just academics. Students with autism spend many taxing hours at school dealing with peers, adults in authority and group expectations, and they may arrive home frazzled and irritable. School is hard work for even the brightest students on the autism spectrum. They often need help navigating the maze of social, sensory, academic and time pressures that school presents. These students need our support and accommodations, but they also need goals that help them learn to fit more comfortably into the world.

The goals described for Mia, Grady and Evan represent some obstacles faced by many highly verbal autistic students in elementary, middle and high school. All three struggle with participating and learning in large and small groups, inhibiting outbursts, interacting successfully with peers and using the executive functions of self-regulation, organization, task initiation and follow-through. They frequently misunderstand figurative or nonverbal communication that comes easily to others. Because of their strengths in other aspects of language and cognition, these deficits in the understanding and use of non-literal, gestural and facial communication may cause some people to think they are deliberately joking or being impertinent. If the errors are seen as naivety or gullibility, teasing is a likely result.

The goals for Mia, Grady and Evan, as described in Chapters 8 and 9, all enhance progress in communication and self-regulation, several goals address peer interaction or increased organization, and each child has at least one goal focused on initiation and follow-through. All of these will be needed for eventual successful employment. Perhaps fairly soon for Evan.

Meeting goals indicates progress but does not preclude later problems. Mia is working on some skills that most children fine-tune in kindergarten. Grady, five years older than Mia and having met all her goals, continues to need help with peer interaction, self-control and self-advocacy. Evan is still working on how his behavior, appearance and tone affect others' perceptions of him. Most of their classmates are progressing faster and more naturally, so presumptions of competency increase. Fragile friendships are difficult to maintain because peers achieve faster developmental growth. Social communication does not come naturally to children on the autism spectrum. They need teaching, practice and to help reach the next level.

It might be tempting to ask "If Mia, Grady and Evan are so bright, why weren't these problems fixed earlier?" Or to say "Their parents should have..." or "Last year's teacher didn't..." But anyone living with a child with autism is likely to have a wide array of issues to deal with and certainly can't do everything. If it is a daily struggle to get your child to accept more than a few foods, do some homework, go to sleep and stay asleep, or transition from pajamas to school clothes in time to catch the bus, you may not have the time and energy to orchestrate play dates, abbreviate monologues and teach organizational skills. Parents can help schools by providing explanations and incentives, but they can't readily control behavior that only happens at school. Teachers can nurture significant progress, but at the end of the school year the child will still be on the autism spectrum.

Other useful skills to teach

Limitations in executive functions such as time management, impulse control, organization of belongings and ideas, transitioning to new tasks or goal planning and follow-through are rampant in middle school. But they are especially obvious among middle and high school students on the autism spectrum. Assistance and practice are vital; these executive functions do not necessarily improve with age. Mia's work on arrival and departure routines, Grady's attempts to use his assignment book and Evan's volunteer work are all steps in developing executive skills and independence.

These children will also need extra help with life skills, social activities, self-advocacy and self-control, some of which are addressed in Chapters 8 and 9. They may need help with hygiene routines, clothing selection and care, calling for a pizza or a haircut, biking, swimming, navigating their communities, driving, learning about laws, negotiating differences and participating in interviews, to name a few.

Social events with peers such as play dates, birthday parties and participation in clubs, activities and sports will require considerable parental assistance. Many children on the autism spectrum avoid participating in sports, perhaps because of factors like poor coordination, low energy, stress about losing or difficulty anticipating the next move of teammates. Encouraging physical activity may be more successful with non-competitive activities like biking and hiking or sports where one can compete for a team but perform as an individual, such as swimming and golf.

Effective self-advocacy requires knowing when, how and from whom to solicit help or accommodations. Some students with autism fall apart emotionally or withdraw and stop participating when confused or overwhelmed. Some even quit jobs because they don't know how to explain that they can't work at the busiest hours or that they don't want to eat with co-workers.

Others may demand or repeatedly request help but be unable to explain what kind of assistance is needed. To locate the problem, start it with him, preferably using a descriptive, fill-in-the-blank format instead of a lot of questions. If you must go over the same information repeatedly, such as the steps of long-division problems, write out the steps and let him read them as he does them.

Some very intelligent children and teens on the autism spectrum seem to be content to remain dependent on their parents. They might even say, as late teenagers, that it is their parents' responsibility to take care of them and may not be especially interested in planning for their future employment. Or they may have unrealistic expectations for career options.

In all areas of learning, measure success by degree of independence, and nurture independence constantly. Keep expecting, and teaching, the next small step and providing incentives if necessary. Expect increased independence to develop gradually and to require consistent effort. It is sometimes easier to encourage a change at notable ages, such as "Now that you are ten years old" or "a teenager" or "a young adult." But the push may have to come from outside the child with autism and may need to include a tangible reward.

Key points on teaching methods

Visual supports

Lists, schedules, cue cards, assignment books, written telephone scripts, recipes, steps to do a math problem and written social narratives and contracts are all examples of visual supports. They make important information clear, direct, reliably the same and available for review. This creates predictability that is very helpful in keeping students on the autism spectrum calm, focused and productive. For students who read easily, the printed word is a strong ally when used in these concrete ways, even if the student's reading comprehension for passages is weak.

Visual supports in the form of social narratives, social contracts and written reminders of things to do or say are used extensively with the goals recommended for Mia, Grady and Evan.

However, autistic students often need adult assistance to use visual supports reliably. A list or narrative lays the groundwork for progress and clarifies what needs to change, but progress requires practice, and a student's willingness to change is often enhanced by incentives. Following are some further thoughts on schedules, social narratives and social contracts.

Schedules

In school, schedules are for everyone. Mia's second-grade teacher may post a list of daily lessons. If not, suggest that it might help Mia and other children if she did. Class rotation schedules will be provided for Grady and Evan and all their classmates. These afford a predictable and comforting framework for the day, and most academically capable students on the autism spectrum readily learn to follow even the sometimes complex and shape-shifting schedules of middle school. Some teachers post the sequence of activities within their individual middle or high school classes, providing even more predictability.

Social narratives

"Social narrative" is used here as a general term for planned, visually presented stories and explanations created by parents and educators to help students with autism regulate behavior, communicate better, interact with peers and live more comfortably and cooperatively. The narratives are written at the child's level of understanding as a way of explaining "This is how it is" or "Something needs to change" in language that will make sense to him or her.

If you can just tell an autistic child a single concrete expectation such as "Boys don't pull girls into their laps in middle school" and he complies thereafter, good. But often more is needed, and ASHA reports an evidence base for the effectiveness of social narratives (Wong *et al.* 2014, p.21).

Social narratives can be used to explain the world, people, a situation or a coming event, usually as an attempt to decrease anxiety and confusion and elicit more appropriate behavior. Carol Gray (2010), with her work on Social Stories™, is the well-known pioneer of this approach. A narrative could help minimize anxiety and constant questioning about an illness, a coming birthday party, a school lockdown, a field trip or a substitute teacher. Narratives of this type may be explanatory and reassuring, and just suggest an appropriate response or course of action.

Or a social narrative might be created to encourage an increase in a positive behavior or to help the student monitor and inhibit a specific undesirable behavior. Often there are lots of behaviors that would be good to change. It is important to let some slide for now and to target one or perhaps group a few that logically go together, such as several aspects of greetings or types of physical aggression. It can be difficult for anyone to modify habits, and even if the student agrees that a requested change is in his best interest, some extrinsic motivation may be needed to assure follow-through.

This is where a social narrative becomes a social contract. In my terms, a social contract is a hybrid of social narrative and reinforcement plan in which you make a deal to tangibly reinforce the changing of a behavior. It is carefully designed and put in writing at the child's comprehension level so that:

+ the child and adults know what to do and expect

+ it can be reviewed for consistency

+ there is a clear expectation of behavior change

+ there is an incentive to motivate the child.

Between a social narrative and a social contract, the major difference—and it can make all the difference—is that you have added a reward.

To create a social narrative or contract, try to work with the child and find solutions together, but have a plan in mind. Discuss his ideas, desired reinforcers and needed accommodations, incorporate them into the contract as much as possible and get his "approval" of the plan. The general plan should explain what needs to change, provide a solution, describe why the change will be better for him and offer an incentive in recognition that it is hard to change a habit.

If he says rewards won't work for him or that he doesn't need the rewards, acknowledge that he doesn't need to accept rewards but that you will still help him make the needed change. Add that you will just keep track of the progress and let him know what he has earned in case he changes his mind. Before starting the plan, and several times in the first week, read the agreement to him calmly, without hurrying and in a reassuring tone. Then you may just let him read it to himself occasionally and he may hear your reassuring rendition in his head.

Putting a social contract in writing is important. The written word often attracts students on the autism spectrum, and writing the contract demonstrates that we have thought seriously about the problem, the student and how to word the narrative. Let the student proofread it for content and mechanical errors. Unlike most oral explanations, the written narrative will stay the same on multiple repetitions. It will be there to refer to if there are disagreements about the content. The aim is to keep all parties calm through multiple exposures and prevent them from becoming agitated or argumentative.

When children have used several different social narratives or plans, it can be helpful to gather them into a reference manual. They may enjoy summary statements for completed plans, such as "I used to get upset when I didn't know how to do something but now I know I can ask for help."

Reinforcement plans

Whether using a single plan that involves reinforcement or a token economy to support several goals as suggested for Grady, be sure that it is precisely and concretely clear how the student earns or fails to earn a point toward the reinforcer. Do not use subjective judgments, even benign and forgiving ones such as "Oh well, you were really trying so I will give you that point." A point is earned because an agreed-upon action happened, or was inhibited as expected, or a product such as a spelling paper was produced, not because someone thinks a student made a good effort. If points are granted on a subjective basis, another adult may withhold a point because there wasn't enough focus and effort. The student with autism is likely to announce, vigorously, that this is unfair.

I do sometimes give bonus points, for reasons that can be specifically described, and that I want the student to repeat, such as:

- ...because you stopped yourself from screaming and asked for help.

- ...because you checked your answers before you passed in the math paper.

- ...because you came back from your break without a reminder from me.

These are clearly labeled as "bonus points," and the actions that precede them are specifically described, concrete actions.

An unearned point can be a big stressor, but it is important for the student to learn that it happens. I never take away earned points; this may be seen as thievery by the student on the autism spectrum. If you really feel the need to impose a consequence, keep it separate from the reinforcement system.

Some key points about reinforcement plans:

+ Focus on a specific issue that the child is capable of changing.

+ Keep language concrete and the expected behavior observable and objective.

+ Put it in writing.

+ Have a strong enough reinforcer, pre-approved by the learner.

+ Follow through.

Modeling and explaining

At this point, modeling is more likely to be a direct request for the child to "try saying it like this." It includes giving Mia or Grady the exact words to say to a classmate in a conflict, demonstrating how to ask a classmate to play or what to say when introducing someone, or showing Evan a more polite alternative when he has been rude. It can also be useful in encouraging more expressive oral reading, better delivery of lines in a play or joke, or more natural-sounding greetings. Because students on the autism spectrum may speak with limited variety of intonation but are often skilled at imitating what they hear, demonstrating appropriate words, intonation and loudness is often effective. If practiced with language that is used frequently, such as greetings, it may generalize and become spontaneous.

Much needs to be explained about social interaction, and the child needs reasons to "try saying it like this" as well as the demonstrations. Reasons such as "It will work better for you," "People will understand it better" or "People will be more willing to help you" may be more meaningful and effective than "It is nicer" or "People will like you better."

When explaining social expectations, try to be as logical and concrete and "autism-friendly" as possible. For example, say that walking quietly in a line keeps children from getting bumped, prevents annoying noises and makes it easy to know what to do. Remember that children with autism can sometimes recite rules without really understanding them. This is especially true if the rules are based on concepts like "respect" and "responsibility" or if they lean away from being literal. When told to "keep your hands to yourself," a young child on the autism spectrum might say "I do! They are stuck to my arms!"

This group of students will also need a lot of explaining of non-literal language and body language. One way to practice is to watch, pause and discuss the words, tone and actions of people in videos.

Reference books are available for idioms and their origins, and you can make your own. Include idioms and metaphors that the child has encountered, with explanations of what they really mean. Make a game out of collecting them, perhaps even deciding to share a favorite snack or activity each time you accumulate 15 new ones.

Emotional support

When everything is going well, don't assume that the child no longer needs support. Mia's regular assistance in grade one was valuable and helped her have a successful school year. But it did not adequately prepare her for independence in the more demanding second grade. If she had practiced being more self-sufficient at the end of first grade, and then had increased adult supervision at the beginning of second grade, the transition could have been smoother for everyone.

Accommodations such as dictation or keyboarding instead of writing by hand, sensory aids such as fidget toys and seat discs, breaks from the classroom and extra adult assistance can all decrease classroom difficulties. It is vital, of course, that the adult assistance comes from people who are calm in the face of rising distress and can apologize when appropriate, avoid raised voices and negative descriptions like "lazy" or "not trying," provide genuine and specific praise, and defuse a stressful situation and revisit it later if necessary. Staying calm when others would be angry may not help the child with autism recognize natural emotional responses, but you can't do everything at once and a crisis is not often a teachable moment.

Behavior

The undesirable behaviors of children in this group are sometimes blamed on their parents. No doubt, there are multiple contributing factors, but I believe that the innate characteristics of autism are the major roots of behavior issues. The behavior section of Chapter 4 describes a lot of these characteristics.

The highly verbal children in this third group are still easily bewildered by idioms, metaphors, sarcasm, group conversation and the meanings of gestures, facial expressions and touch. They are expected to function in mainstream society but frequently find it confusing. Confusion creates anxiety. Anxiety weakens executive, social and general cognitive abilities, and may be expressed as anger or aggression.

Pressure to conform to a group agenda, such as "Do what the class is doing now," are reasonable school expectations but can be problematic when combined with autism's desire to follow its own agenda. Comments like "I'm tired," "It's boring," "I don't like it" or the "automatic No!" are unlikely to elicit empathy from teachers, but may really mean "I don't know how."

Predictable expectations, visual supports, social narratives and contracts, and incentive plans all help students on the autism spectrum maintain acceptable behavior. And in the moment, an adult saying "It's okay, I'll help" can lower anxiety when saying "You must..." could escalate it.

Tracking progress

As always, it is important to know objectively if the students are making progress on their goals. Reports from teachers, parents and even the students themselves can provide some general, though perhaps subjective, information about the impact of the goals and procedures, but you can also collect data.

For Mia's first goal, we have already established that she willingly does the tasks when prompted and that future prompting will be nonverbal. Create a simple chart, dated and with columns for morning arrival and afternoon departure. List the steps she is expected to do and simply use a check mark for the ones she does spontaneously and a "P" for the steps you prompted.

When Mia interviews her classmates, an adult will be with her, so it should be easy to use a similar tracking system to note whether she needed prompts or assistance to initiate the interview, ask the questions, answer her classmates questions, share information and thank the children for coming. Later, you could note her prompted or spontaneous use of the information she learned from the interviews during subsequent conversations with her peers. This data could come from general observation or during a semi-structured activity such as a planned lunch group or social skills group.

Grady's teachers who are helping with the monologue project could use a quick shorthand memo such as "S" for "He stopped before the teacher had to prompt him," "SC" for "He self-corrected and got back on the discussion topic without prompting," "P" for "He stopped when prompted" and "X" for "He kept talking regardless of the pre-arranged prompting."

His progress on completing homework might be reduced to a list indicating whether the assignment was modified, if he wrote it in his assignment book, if he had the needed materials to work on it, if he completed it independently or with help (or not at all), whether he turned it in without a reminder and anything else you want to know. For example, it might be important to know if he spontaneously asked for help, or if his parents or teachers had to notify each other about some glitch.

Since much of the communication work of the children in this group takes place in classrooms and you will be requesting data from busy teachers, it is important to keep the process quick and easy, as with these short lists. More anecdotal information, such as Mia's later conversational use of information from her interviews, is likely to come from teaching assistants or therapists who are working directly with her or with a small group.

For Evan, a "rudeness" checklist could include accepting reminders without arguing, apologizing spontaneously or when prompted, imitating the "better way to say it" or showing no rudeness in a class. In his Goal #3 volunteer job, a teaching assistant or job coach could easily track his performance on the four mini-goals, but we can't expect library staff to do so. However, a library employee might be willing to share a brief oral summary of Evan's skills and areas that could use improvement. Also, ask Evan what he enjoyed about the job, what he would like to change and if any aspects were challenging or stressful.

Comments on notes and narrative summaries make checklists come to life with insights about possible reasons for successes and glitches. One person—the speech/language pathologist perhaps—might write a summary from the checklist data and then confirm its accuracy with the people who had provided the data.

Generalization

Many of the goals for these three students illustrate the beginning of a process of learning a lifelong skill. For example, Mia is improving her ability to complete routines of arrival and departure in a busy environment and to exit calmly from a situation that distresses her. Grady is learning to work as a team member, participate in a discussion without monopolizing it and advocate calmly for himself when upset. Evan is developing an awareness of how his choice of words and tone affect his listeners, and is practicing interactive behaviors appropriate to employment.

Some of their other goals, such as Mia's classmate questions and imitation of exactly what to say to other children, Grady's homework modifications and Evan's structured interviews are currently organized and enabled by adults.

Mastery of this collection of specific goals will not guarantee that Mia, Grady and Evan will use the targeted behaviors in other, similar situations. They will need practice in more environments with increasing expectations of independence, but the experience they gain through these goals should be a strong foundation for faster progress in similar situations.

These goals are not an end, but a strong beginning for communication behaviors with lifelong usefulness for students on the autism spectrum.

What if they are already adults?

Adulthood does not eliminate autism. Finishing high school usually involves loss of mandated support and a simultaneous increase in expected independence. The school and family teams should have been helping the student prepare for this by gradually developing independence over many childhood years.

Whether or not the young person on the autism spectrum goes on to college and perhaps even graduate education, help will probably be needed in adult skills such as driving, dating and living independently.

And eventually, if not immediately, there is the matter of employment. A great number of adults with autism are unemployed or under-employed. Families and often employment coaches and helpful, accommodating employers will be needed to launch young adults on the autism spectrum into meaningful jobs and to help them maintain employment progress.

Independence and employment need to be balanced with outlets for individual "enthusiasms" and social connections. Sometimes, issues of gender identity must be supportively addressed. Reports indicate that gender dysphoria or nonconformity occur more frequently among autistic adolescents than in the general population (Strang *et al.* 2018).

Coming of age with autism is a complex and often challenging life transition with much potential and numerous potholes. It is better navigated with assistance.

Bottom line

Highly verbal children and adults on the autism spectrum often have much knowledge to offer and sometimes express a strong desire to make the world a better place. Difficulties imposed by autism, many of them related to interpersonal communication, may continue to impede their success.

Communication, social behavior and thinking skills are braided together for all of us, with or without autism. The unraveling of one of these strands significantly impacts the others. But growth in each of these areas supports progress in the others and strengthens the whole person. Growth, change and progress can, and should, continue for a lifetime.

Chapter 11

Progress Across
the Spectrum

The premise of this book is that learning functional communication is a factor in helping children all along the autism spectrum become increasingly safe, happy, independent and productive. Communication, interaction, cognition and behavior are all interwoven in this endeavor. Development in any of these areas supports, and depends upon, progress in the others.

Some communication progress for children on the autism spectrum comes from natural growth and development, but much of it requires extra effort from the children, their parents, teachers and therapists. My function as a consultant is to help schools and families address concerns that are not responding to their usual interventions so autistic children can increase their communication and cooperative interaction.

Chapter 11 will illustrate how some of the key methods and supportive techniques I recommended for the nine children in this book are useful at different ability levels and for different concerns. It will mention some other professionals who developed, or use, these and related methods. Because I believe anxiety is the root of many behavioral issues, this chapter will include comments about anxiety from autistic individuals themselves or those who have worked extensively with them.

Three major intervention methods

Let's look at three major methods that were used often in this book and then review other approaches that supported them.

Modeling language and play

In evidence-based practice (EBP), modeling is described as "demonstration of a desired target behavior that results in imitation of the behavior by the learner and that leads to the acquisition of the imitated behavior. This EBP is often combined with other strategies such as prompting and reinforcement" (Wong *et al.* 2014, p.20).

I first encountered modeling in Bloom and Lahey's classic text *Language Development and Language Disorders* (1978) and adapted it over time for echolalia. Barry Prizant (Prizant and Duchan 1981; Prizant and Rydell 1984) was an early influence on my understanding of echolalia, as Carol Westby (1980) was for the language relevance and developmental sequence of play.

Modeling, as I use it across the autism spectrum, evolves with the needs and abilities of the child, and sometimes includes aspects of prompting, scripting and reinforcement.

Visual supports

Wong *et al.* (2014, p.22) describe visual supports as:

Any visual display that supports the learner engaging in a desired behavior or skills independent of prompts. Examples of visual supports include pictures, written words, objects within the environment, arrangement of the environment or visual boundaries, schedules, maps, labels, organization systems, and timelines.

Schedules, object and picture systems for expressive communication, "wait" symbols, written narratives, contracts, cue cards, reminders and lists are all examples of visual supports used in this book. Using

American Sign Language along with speech is another valuable visual strategy. Visual supports contribute greatly to making learning more errorless and to decreasing the need for adult prompts.

Linda Hodgdon (1995) has written and presented extensively about visual support systems. She also refers to them as "visual tools" or "visual strategies." Carol Gray's Social Stories™ (2010) introduced another important visually based strategy to the communication education of autistic children. And Lori Frost and Andy Bondy's Picture Exchange Communication System (PECS) (2002) made picture-based communication a deliberately interactive process. Wong *et al.* (2014, p.21) list PECS specifically as an evidence-based practice. The work of all these people has had a tremendous international impact on improving communication for people on the autism spectrum.

Incentive plans and reinforcement

Reinforcement refers to "an event, activity, or other circumstance occurring after a learner engages in a desired behavior that leads to the increased occurrence of the behavior in the future" (Wong *et al.* 2014, p.21).

Reinforcement is a major premise of the work of B.F. Skinner (1957) and an integral part of instruction via Applied Behavior Analysis (ABA) and related programs (Barbera 2007; Lovaas 1987; Rogers, Dawson and Vismara 2012). As seen multiple times for the children in this book, an incentive plan may include a behavior plan, such as a social contract, and a reinforcer or token economy.

I believe that reinforcement is a very important, often vital, part of intervention with students on the autism spectrum. It is usually but not always effective. To improve the likelihood of success, be sure to:

- Match the plan to the child's cognitive level. Arnie and Darius may not understand an expectation not to hit or throw things, but they will recognize that they are rewarded for putting a piece in a puzzle or imitating an action. They can also fairly quickly learn to accept five tokens as reinforcers before being given the actual reward.

+ Be specific and concrete. Terek, Mia, Grady and Evan may not know the details of "being responsible" or "showing respect," but they can learn to inhibit saying certain words at school or practice better ways to speak to adults or peers or finish a paper and check their work.

+ Keep it factual and objective. Write down the agreements and follow through on them as written, without subjective judgements such as withholding a reward because the task took too long or the student's "attitude" wasn't good.

Modeling, visual supports and reinforcement for the children in this book

These three methods were used frequently in previous chapters to meet goals for the nine children along the autism spectrum.

Pre-symbolic communication and emerging speech group

Rebecca's teachers consistently model the names of her free-choice toys and her scheduled activities to enhance her comprehension/receptive language. It is unlikely that she will say the words, although that would be wonderful.

Her schedule and choice board are strong visual tools that are allowing her to understand actions and expectations that she cannot comprehend from words alone. Her object symbols are being used as a bridge to recognizing pictures, to minimize behavioral issues at the end of her walks, and as hallway navigational aids. The careful visual/tactile arrangement of her table task items helps Rebecca complete the work more independently. Even the practice of using linear schedules and circular choice boards helps her "see" the difference between an expectation and a choice.

Although Rebecca appears willing and content to participate in these school activities now that she understands them, it would probably not have been possible to maintain her attention and develop cooperation without reinforcers important to her. Carefully dispensed cheese balls have been essential to her progress.

Like Rebecca, Arnie hears single words modeled repeatedly during his receptive vocabulary practice and matching or sorting activities. The present goal is for him to understand the words, but there is definite intent that he will also someday say them.

His picture exchange boards for requesting, the "wait" symbol, and the matching or similar objects and pictures shown to him while practicing "Give me the..." and when matching or sorting are all forms of visual support.

When making a request by giving someone a symbol, he is naturally reinforced by getting the item he asked for, but he definitely needs deliberate reinforcers, often with ketchup, to focus on new learning.

Darius has play skills, words and meaningful sounds modeled for him in semi-structured play sessions, directed table work and daily-life routines, including those times when he makes a request through nonverbal actions. Visual support comes from his schedule and the materials he uses for picture exchange and for requesting by pointing.

He is also working on imitating speech on request, for which strong reinforcers are given. This may help increase his response to modeled speech in less structured activities. During table work, as he becomes more cooperative and willing to participate because he enjoys the activities, extrinsic reinforcement can be decreased.

Atypical language group

Because Lucas echoes speech readily, he is especially responsive to modeling. The problem is that he imitates what he hears whether or not it is an appropriate model for him. Therefore, modeling for him is built on minimizing questions and pronouns, and matching language to his perspective on events.

Since he is hyperlexic, his visual strategies can use words more than pictures. Lucas enjoys following a schedule of printed words, benefits from seeing name tags as he learns to greet people by name, and can practice directives for the "Everybody" game by reading them off cue cards. The hand-to-chest "I" cue is a visual/tactile strategy that is an essential part of intervention for Lucas.

Natural reinforcement of obtaining a requested item or action, avoiding undesirables and maintaining an interaction are often sufficient to keep Lucas attentive.

Seth benefits from hearing modeled language from the third person in his yes/no practice or his teachers showing and telling him about locational concepts. And the scripts he hears for his personal care routines and travel routes are important models for him to memorize and use independently.

Because he is blind, his "visual" supports are tactile. They include his brailled "No chanting" reminder, the arrangement, symbols and "All done" card of his independent work, and even the separate sorting piles for learning "yes/no" and "he/she." Reinforcement is offered for the "No chanting" plan and as needed for other learning.

For Terek, modeling now takes the form of specific direction about what he should say and the intonation he should use. At this point, it might better be called "scripting," an evidence-based practice described by Wong et al. (2014, p.21) as "a verbal and/or written description about a specific skill or situation that serves as a model for the learner."

Terek is given specific suggestions of things to say to Arielle and to students who annoy him. These instructions are made visible in written social narratives and contracts. He works on question forms by initially reading them, and the structure of his independent work folder helps him stay focused and transition between tasks. Terek should have a schedule that provides predictability but also has a strategy for showing changes, and he should be learning to follow it with minimal prompting.

His social contracts include reinforcers for using positive behaviors and inhibiting negative ones. These social contracts, and many other interventions in this book, are examples of another evidence-based practice, functional communication training or "replacement of interfering behavior that has a communication function with more appropriate communication that accomplishes the same function" (Wong et al. 2014, p.20).

Advanced language with gaps group

For Mia, adult and peer models of "good game" are part of her plan for accepting losing a game, and adults demonstrate the exact words and tone she can use for invitations, apologies or explanations to peers.

Her visual tools are written lists, narratives and cue cards related to arrival and departure routines, winning and losing, and needing a break. She also has a written script to guide her classmate interviews. Reinforcement for following her different plans is generally in the form of short privileges.

Modeling exact words, timing and intonation can also help Grady deal with peer interactions or learn to tell jokes more effectively. He has written communication through multiple social contracts, his problem page, steps for completing math problems and the arrangement of his assignment book. Reinforcement is built into his social contracts and combined into a token economy.

Evan has direct practice in imitating a model through the "better way to say it" part of his rudeness goal. He has visual supports such as written explanations and contracts, listed expectations for his library responsibilities and notes to highlight or copy. Extrinsic reinforcers are included in some social contracts through an unobtrusive token economy.

Supportive methods and techniques

Modeling, visual supports and positive reinforcement can be used in many ways to support cooperative behavior while developing more effective communication. Other techniques which work well with them include the following.

"Just start"

Just starting an activity helps the child by getting past the stress of transition and the alarm of "I don't know how!" When I recommend that adults "just start" an activity with a child on the autism spectrum, I don't mean forcing him to do it. I mean showing how it is done, often by doing it yourself with no pressure on the child to respond. Put the first piece in the puzzle yourself, start naming a few pictures in the book, sort the first few colors and give yourself the reinforcer, describe the steps as you do the first math problem, start reading the passage and say "This is important" as you underline a key point. For young children, who might just dash off and not even see your demonstration, you may also be including some hand-over-hand prompting of a simple step and quickly following up with a treat. I find this technique to be less stressful and more successful than crossing your arms and saying, "Tell me when you are ready to work." Often, once the student realizes that he can do the task or that you will be helping, he is able to begin.

Nonverbal prompting

Children on the autism spectrum can become very dependent on prompts, and physical prompts have generally been found to be easier to fade than verbal prompts. I've observed that autistic students will often respond as if a verbal prompt is an essential part of a task and wait for the prompt even when not needing it. My advice is to prompt, or help, as much as you have to and as little as you can get away with, since the goal is always independence.

At times it is very helpful to have a second adult do the physical prompting silently while you interact with the child. Children are easily confused by two people talking at once, and a silent prompter can help the child to respond while focusing on the speaker. But this luxury is not always available, and everything recommended here can be and has been done by one adult.

Visual supports often decrease the need for adult prompts.

Errorless learning

The development of errorless learning and examples of its use are described in an article by Mueller, Palkovic and Maynard (2007). Errorless learning refers to teaching procedures that may not eliminate, but certainly reduce the chance that children will make errors in a learning task. It is an important part of many educational programs for autism. I often describe errorless learning as "teaching, not testing" and find that it eliminates a lot of confusion and frustration for children on the autism spectrum.

Structured and natural context teaching

Some teaching can be done in a natural context such as modeling language during daily routines or in combination with the modeling of play skills. Teachable moments include explaining the meaning of figurative language or a behavior the child has noticed. Parents often use car travel as an opportunity for descriptions, discussions and verbal games.

Naturalistic intervention is included as an evidence-based practice, described by Wong *et al.* (2014, p.20) as:

> Intervention strategies that occur within the typical setting/ activities/routines in which the learner participates. Teachers/ service providers establish the learner's interest in a learning event through arrangement of the setting/activity/routine, provide necessary support for the learner to engage in the targeted behavior, elaborate on the behavior when it occurs, and/or arrange natural consequences for the targeted behavior or skills.

Often, however, more structured, directed teaching situations are needed to gain and maintain the student's attention and to clarify the information being taught. Most of regular education occurs in a structured teaching environment. ABA programs contain a lot of individual directed instruction. For all children, autistic or not, both types of instruction are essential.

Communicate clearly and directly

If you want to maximize the child's chances of understanding, use simple unambiguous language when the situation is urgent or confusing. This could mean saying "Stop! Sit down!" instead of "Watch out for the cars!" to a young child running toward the road, explaining behavioral objectives in a written narrative or putting a figure of speech into literal terms for a teenager. You can joke, play with words and expand vocabulary and verbal knowledge when all is calm, but stay near the child's base level of comprehension when he is anxious or stressed.

Accept anxiety as a part of autism

Anxiety may not be part of the diagnostic criteria for autism, but it is often there. Here is what a few professionals and people on the autism spectrum have said:

Temple Grandin (Grandin and Johnson 2005), who famously both lives with and explains autism, says:

> Fear is a horrible problem for people with autism—fear *and* anxiety. (p.191)

> Autistic people have so much natural fear and anxiety—I'm almost comfortable saying it's universal. (p.192)

> In my own case, overwhelming anxiety hit at puberty... I was in a constant daily state of emergency. (p.193)

Other authors on the autism spectrum add:

> Like a lot of people on the autism spectrum, I have suffered with chronic anxiety for a long time. Simple things like just walking into

cafes and bars, being around people or walking down the street become daunting, challenging tasks. (Jackson 2016, p.182)

I am always vulnerable to anxiety. Both good things and bad things can bring it on. Parties, shopping, playing on the computer are all as anxiety provoking to me as traffic jams, long lines and bad news. I've been on and off various medications to deal with anxiety, but even when the anxieties are numbed, the reality is that I always sense I'm but one step ahead of the anxiety avalanche. (Willey 2003, pp.180–181)

Everywhere I looked, there were threats. The kids around me were unpredictable. Teachers were just waiting to pounce on me and punish me for fun. Strangers were worse—they lurked outside the school, waiting to kidnap unwary kids. Whom could I trust? It seemed like my parents were safe, and maybe a few kids, but that was about it. With all that, you might think I was a scared little kid, but I really wasn't. I was just cautious. Cautious and wary. And prepared. (Robison 2011, p.73)

Whether or not anxiety leads to behavioral problems, Tony Attwood points out its debilitating effects on people:

One of the problems faced by children with Asperger's syndrome who use their intellect rather than intuition to succeed in some social situations is that they may be in an almost constant state of alertness and anxiety, leading to risk of mental and physical exhaustion. (Attwood 2007, p.29)

And Barbara Bissonnette still encounters anxiety and its fallout in her employment coaching for adults on the autism spectrum, saying:

Anxiety drives impulsive actions that may lead, ultimately, to job loss. (Bissonnette 2015, p.49)

Education to develop competencies, especially in communication, helps to lessen anxiety, behavioral disruptions and especially emotional meltdowns. So does another evidence-based practice called antecedent-based intervention, which involves "arrangement of events or circumstances that precede the occurrence of an interfering behavior and [are] designed to lead to the reduction of the behavior" (Wong *et al.* 2014, p.20).

I call this "prevention" and it includes many of the techniques suggested here, such as predictable schedules, "just start," errorless learning, clear, direct communication, visual supports, goals matched to development and carefully timed reinforcement. It may also mean not eating in the cafeteria, going outdoors before the fire drill, buying several pairs of the same exact pants, or putting a lifejacket on a little girl by her wading pool so she can't remove her bathing suit in the back yard. Parents and teachers become very adept at taking preventative measures to minimize meltdowns even while they are working steadily on progress.

Manage meltdowns

Despite everyone's best efforts at prevention and education, there will still be emotional meltdowns at school, home and/or in the community. Then the goal is to recover and move on as smoothly as possible. Some things that help:

• **Support:** The calm, helpful adult, someone the student feels will keep him safe, is a tremendous asset. Believe and convey "I'm sorry you're upset. I'm here to help."

• **Silence:** This means minimizing language, noise and confusion. Total silence would probably be impossible to produce, but don't say much. This child is easily confused even when calm, and lots of words now will make things worse.

• **Sensory:** Aim for accommodations that add comfort or remove the stressors that fuel the meltdown. Quiet and change of location, dim lights or a place to retreat often speed recovery. This is not the time to introduce something new or hug someone who resists touch.

• **Sameness:** Try to provide something familiar and non-taxing for the child to latch on to mentally. For some, just starting a familiar activity will help the student re-engage but be sure it reflects an easy expectation right now and does not include an immediate return to the scene of the explosion.

Be a team

Work together to develop and meet functional goals and then do it again.

Raising and educating any child, but especially one on the autism spectrum, is a marathon, not a sprint.

There should always be progress, with some setbacks and plateaus, but the speed of progress will vary. Expect these variations and keep going. Sail when you can, and if there's no wind, row.

References

American Psychiatric Association (APA) (2013) *Diagnostic and Statistical Manual of Mental Disorders, Fifth Edition*. Arlington, VA: American Psychiatric Association.

American Speech-Language-Hearing Association (ASHA) (2005) "Evidence-Based Practice in Communication Disorders." Accessed on 12/5/2019 at www.asha.org/policy/ps2005-00221.htm.

Attwood, T. (2007) *The Complete Guide to Asperger's Syndrome*. London: Jessica Kingsley Publishers.

Barbera, M.L. (2007) *The Verbal Behavior Approach: How to Teach Children with Autism and Related Disorders*. London: Jessica Kingsley Publishers.

Bissonnette, B. (2015) *Helping Adults with Asperger's Syndrome Get and Stay Hired: Career Coaching Strategies for Professionals and Parents of Adults on the Autism Spectrum*. London: Jessica Kingsley Publishers.

Bloom, L. and Lahey, M. (1978) *Language Development and Language Disorders*. New York, NY: John Wiley & Sons.

Eckenrode, L., Fennell, P. and Hearsey, K. (2003) *Tasks Galore*. Raleigh, NC: Tasks Galore Publishing.

Frost, L. and Bondy, A. (2002) *The Picture Exchange Communication System Training Manual*. Newark, DE: Pyramid Educational Products.

Grandin, T. and Johnson, C. (2005) *Animals in Translation*. New York, NY: Harcourt.

Gray, C. (2010) *The New Social Story Book*. Arlington TX: Future Horizons.

Hodgdon, L.A. (1995) *Visual Strategies for Improving Communication*. Troy, MI: QuirkRoberts Publishing.

Jackson, L. (2016) *Sex, Drugs and Asperger's Syndrome (ASD): A User Guide to Adulthood*. London: Jessica Kingsley Publishers.

Lovaas, O.I. (1987) "Behavioral treatment and normal educational and intellectual functioning in young autistic children." *Journal of Consulting and Clinical Psychology* 55, 1, 3–9.

Mesibov, G.B., Shea, V. and Schopler, E. (2005) *The TEACCH Approach to Autism Spectrum Disorders.* New York, NY: Springer.

Millar, D.C., Light, J.C. and Schlosser, R.W. (2006) "The impact of augmentative and alternative communication intervention on the speech production of individuals with developmental disabilities: A research review." *Journal of Speech and Hearing Research 49,* 2, 248–264.

Mueller, M.M., Palkovic, C.M. and Maynard, C.S. (2007) "Errorless learning: Review and practical applications for teaching children with pervasive developmental disorders." *Psychology in the Schools 44,* 7, 691–700.

Prizant, B.M. and Duchan, J.F. (1981) "The functions of immediate echolalia in autistic children." *Journal of Speech and Hearing Disorders 46,* 3, 241–249.

Prizant, B.M. and Rydell, P.J. (1984) "Analysis of functions of delayed echolalia in autistic children." *Journal of Speech and Hearing Research 27,* 2, 183–192.

Prizant, B. with Fields-Meyer, T. (2015) *Uniquely Human: A Different Way of Seeing Autism.* New York, NY: Simon and Schuster.

Robison, J.E. (2011) *Be Different: Adventures of a Free-Range Aspergian.* New York, NY: Crown Archetype.

Rogers, S.J., Dawson, G. and Vismara, L.A. (2012) *An Early Start for Your Child with Autism.* New York, NY: The Guilford Press.

Skinner, B.F. (1957) *Verbal Behavior.* Englewood Cliffs, NJ: Prentice-Hall.

Strang, J.F., Meagher, H., Kenworthy, L., DeVries, A.L.C. *et al.* (2018) "Initial clinical guidelines for co-occurring autism spectrum disorder and gender dysphoria or incongruence in adolescents." *Journal of Clinical Child and Adolescent Psychology 47,* 1, 105–115.

Westby, C. (1980) "Assessment of cognitive and language abilities through play." *Language Speech and Hearing Services in Schools 11,* 3, 154–168.

Willey, L.H. (2003) "When the Thunder Roars." In L.H. Willey (ed.) *Asperger Syndrome in Adolescence: Living with the Ups, the Downs and Things in Between.* London: Jessica Kingsley Publishers.

Wong, C., Odom, S.L., Hume, K., Cox, A.W. *et al.* (2014) *Evidence-Based Practices for Children, Youth, and Young Adults with Autism Spectrum Disorder.* Chapel Hill: The University of North Carolina, Frank Porter Graham Child Development Institute, Autism Evidence-Based Practice Review Group. Accessed on 12/5/2019 at https:// autismpdc.fpg.unc.edu/sites/autismpdc.fpg.unc.edu/files/2014-EBP-Report.pdf.

Index